P9-DER-188

PRAISE FOR

the mindful vegan

"*The Mindful Vegan* isn't just a book, it's Lani Muelrath herself. In the years I've known her, I have always admired how remarkably present she is in every moment. This book is a gift to those of us who desire the same presence of mind and shows us, in bite-sized steps, how to attain that with ease and joy."

**—Miyoko Schinner, author of *Artisan Vegan Cheese*
and *The Homemade Vegan Pantry* and founder of Miyoko's Kitchen**

"Read, implement, transform...and then pass along the magic! This book can heal you."

**—Kathy Freston, *New York Times* bestselling author
of *Quantum Wellness***

"At this moment in history, more people than ever before have the freedom to consciously choose what we eat. Science clearly shows us that eating whole plant foods is the optimum dietary choice, and it turns out that what's good for our health is also good for our planet and our fellow creatures. Eating a vegan diet is a win-win-win! But that doesn't mean it's always easy. In connecting the ancient practice of mindfulness with the business of nourishing ourselves, Lani Muelrath's *The Mindful Vegan* offers a powerful tool to support readers in making the choice, each day, to live a more compassionate and healthy life."

**—John Mackey, cofounder and CEO of Whole Foods Market
and coauthor of *The Whole Foods Diet***

"*The Mindful Vegan* calls us to pay attention to the profound impacts of our food choices and encourages us to act in alignment with our humanity. This enlivening book inspires us to live with passion and purpose, and gives us the tools to make more mindful choices that are good for ourselves, other animals and the planet. Think about it, as *The Mindful Vegan* asks us, if we can live well without causing unnecessary harm, why wouldn't we? Highly recommended."

—Gene Baur, cofounder and president of Farm Sanctuary and author of *Living the Farm Sanctuary Life*

"Lani takes conscious living up a notch with this beautiful guide whose ripple effects extend far and wide. Long before you finish, you will have a much deeper connection to your own compassion— and a much broader understanding of what it means to live mindfully."

—Colleen Patrick-Goudreau, bestselling author of *The 30-Day Vegan Challenge* and host of the *Food for Thought* podcast

"Mindfulness is probably the most important practice we can ever undertake. The more we are able to be mindful, or present, the more we are able to feel authentically connected with ourselves and others. The ability to be present is at the heart of all healthy relationships: with other humans, with nonhuman beings, with the planet, and with ourselves. In this wonderful book, Lani Muelrath explains, with compassion and clarity, how you can eat and live more mindfully—and thus how you can transform your life."

—Dr. Melanie Joy, author of *Why We Love Dogs, Eat Pigs, and Wear Cows* and *Beyond Beliefs: A Guide to Improving Relationships and Communication for Vegans, Vegetarians, and Meat Eaters*

"These thirty life-shifting days with Lani Muelrath link sustenance with silence, nutrition with attention. You'll finish this book knowing that you've made peace with food and you've made friends with yourself."

—Victoria Moran, author *Main Street Vegan* and director of the Main Street Vegan Academy

"I absolutely LOVE this book. If your relationship with food has been a bit of a rocky road, it is a must read. Lani Muelrath brilliantly guides readers through a personal exploration that engages our senses and sensibilities. She provides a blueprint for mindfulness that establishes an honest, joy-filled connection with food, and with our bodies. Her goals are simple—health and healing for individuals; compassion and peace for the world. What a beautiful gift to us all."

—Brenda Davis, RD, coauthor of
Becoming Vegan

"*The Mindful Vegan* is a heartfelt approach to transforming life one bite at a time. Being conscious of a decision to honor your health, the life of animals, and our precious planet is the focus of this excellent book and can be a path to elevating the quality of our daily existence. A life with purpose is a key step to fulfillment and *The Mindful Vegan* is the key that can unlock that precious treasure chest of a meaningful and healthy life."

—Joel Kahn, MD, FACC, clinical professor of medicine (cardiology) and director at The Kahn Center for Cardiac Longevity and author of *The Whole Heart Solution*

"As we see increasing numbers of people questioning the official stories of Western culture, we're also benefitting from the ancient wisdom traditions of the East. With *The Mindful Vegan,* Lani Muelrath provides us with a rich program of helpful insights that illuminate two mutually supporting pillars of this wisdom: mindfulness and vegan living. As a Zen monk in Korea in the 1980s, I was blessed to drink from this well of wisdom, and am delighted that Lani's new book helps provide this crucial and missing piece to our culture today. *The Mindful Vegan* can transform your life, and would also make a terrific gift for virtually anyone. Recommended!"

—Will Tuttle, PhD, author of *The World Peace Diet*,
visionary educator, musician, and presenter

"*The Mindful Vegan* is a groundbreaking and compassionate guide that connects mindfulness practice to the larger ecological and health benefits of veganism. Its 30-day plan offers a beautifully thought-out approach to learning mindfulness that will help you investigate your relationship to food, dieting and self-care. This book could change your life (whether or not you are vegan)! Plus, I can't wait to try the recipes."

—Diana Winston, director of mindfulness education at UCLA
Mindful Awareness Research Center and coauthor of
Fully Present: The Science, Art, and Practice of Mindfulness

"Lani, you have done it again–with your latest book *The Mindful Vegan*, you have created an evidence-based pathway to experiencing deeper joy, better health, longer life, and a greater chance for planetary survival. You draw out the best in us: courage, commitment, compassion, and choices of how to use our fork and knife with greater wisdom and mindfulness."

—Hans Diehl, DrHSc, clinical professor of preventive medicine
at Loma Linda University, founder of CHIP and
Lifestyle Medicine Institute, and coauthor of *Health Power*

"As a clinician, researcher, and teacher who works on a daily basis to help people change their stress and emotional eating habits, I've seen firsthand how powerful mindfulness can be in the food arena. *The Mindful Vegan* is full of heart, accessibility, and practicality."

—Judson Brewer, MD, PhD, associate professor of medicine
and psychiatry and director of research at the Center
for Mindfulness, UMASS Medical School, creator of Eat Right Now,
and author of *The Craving Mind*

"Mindfulness is an incredibly powerful practice essential for becoming the best version of you. With Lani Muelrath's *The Mindful Vegan*, you now have a brilliant, beautiful, and practical guide with over 30 days of tools and techniques for unlocking the door to the blessing that is mindfulness."

—Marco Borges, exercise physiologist and *New York Times*
bestselling author of *The 22 Day Revolution*

"Warm and wise, informed by science and experience, *The Mindful Vegan* is a welcome invitation and map to connection with our minds and bodies, with others, and with the present moment. Watch for delight arising as you take this life-changing journey with Lani Muelrath as your skillful guide— and again when you discover the vegan recipes included after day 30."

—Patti Breitman, cofounder of Dharma Voices for Animals
and coauthor of *Even Vegans Die*

"Lani Muelrath has been a source of information and inspiration for radiant health through plant based eating. *The Mindful Vegan* is a beacon of conscious eating, healthy living, and caring for the planet—with a 30-day plan that will set you on the path of transforming your life."

—Suzy Amis Cameron, founder of Plant Power Task Force

"The teachings found in *The Mindful Vegan* are life's secret weapon to reduce your anxiety, stress, anger, and fear and replace those negative emotions with peace, clarity, happiness, and optimism. Practicing mindfulness has been especially helpful for me since going vegan as I've been able to navigate through the nightmare I woke up to with patience and understanding instead of resentment and bitterness. It's helped me come from an encouraging and compassionate place when advocating to others and is a vital piece to the puzzle in making this world a more peaceful place, and I am glad to see mindfulness and vegan living brought together so brilliantly in this book. It will change, for the better, your experience of living."

—James Aspey, speaker and vegan advocate

"In over 40 years of conducting clinical research, my colleagues and I have shown that a whole foods plant-based diet (naturally low in refined carbs and fat), along with meditation/yoga, exercise, and social support (love & intimacy) can reverse the progression of the most common chronic diseases. The more illnesses we study, and the more underlying biological mechanisms we examine, the more reasons we have to explain why these lifestyle changes are so powerful and how quickly they may occur. *The Mindful Vegan* eloquently describes why, and how.

—Dean Ornish, MD, Clinical Professor of Medicine, UCSF, Founder & President, Preventive Medicine Research Institute and author of six books, all bestsellers

the mindful vegan

the mindful vegan

A 30-Day Plan
for Finding Health, Balance, Peace, and Happiness

Lani Muelrath, MA

BENBELLA BOOKS, INC.
Dallas, TX

Copyright © 2017 by Lani Muelrath

"Light Bulb" by Jose Moya from Noun Project is licensed under CC BY 3.0.
"Lotus" by Karthik Srinivas from Noun Project is licensed under CC BY 3.0.
"Meditation" by Karthik Srinivas from Noun Project is licensed under CC BY 3.0.
"Volume Control" by IconDots from Noun Project is licensed under CC BY 3.0.

All rights reserved. No part of this book may be used or reproduced in any manner whatsoever
without written permission except in the case of brief quotations embodied in critical articles or reviews.

BenBella
BenBella Books, Inc.
10440 N. Central Expressway, Suite 800
Dallas, TX 75231
www.benbellabooks.com
Send feedback to feedback@benbellabooks.com

Printed in the United States of America
10 9 8 7 6 5 4 3 2

Library of Congress Cataloging-in-Publication Data:

Names: Muelrath, Lani, author.
Title: The mindful vegan : a 30-day plan for finding health, balance, peace,
and happiness / by Lani Muelrath, MA.
Description: Dallas, TX : BenBella Books, Inc., [2017] | Includes
bibliographical references and index.
Identifiers: LCCN 2017019828 (print) | LCCN 2017030014 (ebook) | ISBN
9781944648480 (electronic) | ISBN 9781944648473 (trade cloth : alk. paper)
Subjects: LCSH: Vegetarianism. | Veganism. | Food habits--Psychological
aspects. | Vegetarian cooking.
Classification: LCC RM236 (ebook) | LCC RM236 .M84 2017 (print) | DDC
613.2/62--dc23
LC record available at https://lccn.loc.gov/2017019828

Editing by Vy Tran
Copyediting by Nicole Brugger-Dethmers
Proofreading by Michael Fedison and Cape Code Compositors, Inc.
Indexing by Clive Pyne
Text design and composition by John Reinhardt Book Design
Front cover design by Connie Gabbert
Jacket design by Sarah Avinger
Author photo by LUMI Photography
Printed by Lake Book Manufacturing

Distributed to the trade by Two Rivers Distribution, an Ingram brand
www.tworiversdistribution.com

Special discounts for bulk sales (minimum of 25 copies) are available.
Please contact Aida Herrera at aida@benbellabooks.com.

For all the wild places, and dear Greg who has taken me to them

For all the open spaces of our lands, our oceans, and our hearts

May all be healthy, happy, and safe

Mindfulness is probably the most important practice we can ever undertake. The more we are able to be mindful, or present, the more we are able to feel authentically connected with ourselves and "others." The ability to be present is at the heart of all healthy relationships: with other humans, with nonhuman beings, with the planet, and with ourselves. When we are present, we relate to all aspects of our lives—including our eating habits—with greater awareness, compassion, and health.

—DR. MELANIE JOY, author of *Why We Love Dogs, Eat Pigs, and Wear Cows,* and *Beyond Beliefs: A Guide to Improving Relationships and Communication for Vegans, Vegetarians, and Meat Eaters*, founder and president, Beyond Carnism

contents

PART THREE

recipes

breakfast

dressing and sauces

salads and savory main dishes

sweet finishes

foreword

THIS BOOK IS DESPERATELY NEEDED and long overdue. Because when it comes to food choices nowadays, "mindful" is just about the last word you might think of. Turn on the television and half the commercials are for burgers, pizza, and snack foods, while the other half are pitching medications to undo the effects of the unhealthful foods we're eating. With most adults weighing more than they would like, and many facing heart disease, diabetes, and other diet-related problems, we are clearly not where we need to be.

But what does mindfulness mean?

To some people, it simply means paying attention. At dinnertime, for example, rather than nibbling while we watch television, it pays to be aware of the flavors of the foods we're eating and to notice when we've had enough. Being mindful of our food choices means we'll be less likely to overeat and more likely to recognize how foods affect us. We will be less drawn to those "addicting" foods—you know which ones attract you—and more likely to make healthful choices.

And mindfulness extends beyond mealtime. Meditation, yoga, and other stress-taming techniques help us get in tune with ourselves and the world around us. They help us rebound from the stresses of the day and be on a better path for the challenges to come.

But mindfulness is more than paying attention while you eat and using exercises to tame distractions and stress. It is a way of being in charge. Instead of feeling like a pinball bouncing from one thing to another, we are making smart decisions.

However, a word of caution. Mindfulness is not the same as *escape*. It does not mean retiring to a secluded refuge for a life of uninterrupted bliss. When you are truly mindful of the consequences of food choices, you will come to see the dangers that unhealthful foods can pose to you or your loved ones. You will reflect on those around you and will see how food habits—healthful or otherwise—are passed from parent to child. Becoming mindful can mean being concerned about the fact that Americans now eat *one million animals every hour* and contribute more to climate change than all the cars, planes, and all other forms of transport combined. It can mean thinking globally and seeing how bad food habits spread from country to country, carrying health problems with them. Being mindful means wanting to jump in and change things.

When we see the surprisingly large role that food choices play in our lives, the issues might seem a bit daunting.

But take heart. We can draw a helpful lesson from those who fought for peace a century ago. As the world emerged from the wreckage of the World War I, far-sighted people sought a new way to solve conflicts. Establishing the League of Nations and later the United Nations, they endeavored to bring humankind to a new level of discourse. Whether their efforts will prove successful over the long term is anyone's guess. But here is the point: When one of the League of Nation's framers was asked, "Are you optimistic?" he replied, "I'm am not optimistic or pessimistic. I am determined."

The same attitude applies to tackling food issues. We do not need to be optimistic or pessimistic about our ability to get animals off the plate, solve climate problems, and help people get healthier. We simply need to do what we can.

Wow! That's heady stuff, you are no doubt thinking. Well, don't worry. For now, our goal is not to solve the world's problems or to jump into serious philosophy. Rather, we're just going to get ourselves in balance, becoming clear-headed and awake to the world around us. But I raise these issues to show that mindfulness can be powerful.

And we'll start easily. Just a minute of practice on day 1—that's right, just one minute. And two minutes on day 2, and so on. You'll see how incredibly doable it is.

Along the way, you'll feel confident, and every day you'll be stronger, whether you are tackling a few unwanted pounds, a more serious health issue, or the state of the world.

Lani Muelrath will be your guide. She knows what she is talking about, and if you trust her method and put it to work, you will see how simple it can be. It works. You'll love it, and it will help you be the person you want to be.

—Neal Barnard, MD, FACC

introduction

ASTRONOMERS HAVE BEEN on a celestial treasure hunt for a certain undiscovered planet since early 2014. As of this writing no one has actually seen this mystery planet, temporarily dubbed Planet Nine, though scientists have good reason to believe it is lurking in the distant reaches of our solar system. Its presence is the only explanation they can find for the behavior of several other heavenly bodies nearby. The proximity of a large planet—bigger than planet Earth, beyond the reaches of Neptune—would account for their orbital patterns, their uniform tilt, and the fact that this field of icy objects and debris never ventures outside of a specific range. All signs point to a planetary tug—"as if they're being pulled by something big."[1]

In like fashion, our habits—reactions of thought, word and deed, moods, and mind frames—are the orbiting objects of our personal inner mental mass. Our demeanor and conduct reflect our inner condition. We may be quite familiar with our reactions and how we deal with likes and dislikes. Yet it is clear to us that some of these well-worn patterns—the objects and debris orbiting our personal planet, if you will—are getting in the way of our greater happiness. So we try to change our habits: eat better, get more exercise, be more patient and kind, and be a better example for the change we want to see in the world. We often find that our attempts to change these outer expressions—trying to alter the orbit of, eject, or otherwise manipulate our habits—is difficult if not impossible. It can feel like trying to push the moon out of its path around Earth, beyond the bounds of possibility due to the laws of physics. After all, the only way the moon might be nudged from its earthly orbit would be if something about Earth herself were to change, resulting in an altered orbital pathway for our moon as a natural consequence.

It is the same with us. Like Planet Nine, though we may not see the origins of our behaviors, the influence of our mental mass is there just the same. And despite our belief that we know ourselves best, research tells us that we have multiple blind spots when it comes to understanding our patterns of thinking, feeling, and behaving. When compassion, generosity, love, and other thoughts and actions spontaneously arise from our innate qualities of kindness and caring, they bring positive results. Yet these blind spots—gaps in our self-knowledge—can also have profound negative consequences. They can show up as automaticity: reactive behaviors, thinking loops, mindless and stress eating, problems with interpersonal communications, anxiety, and unskillful decision-making. These can cause a great deal of confusion, frustration, sadness, and personal misery.[2]

In other words, there's a high cost to this disconnect. If you've ever felt frustrated by finding yourself mired in a familiar negative pattern, or baffled by repeat behaviors in spite of your designs to do otherwise, you are experiencing automaticity in action. At lunch the person at the table next to you digs into a big slab of meat, rattling your sensibilities. You arrive home after a busy day and find yourself up to your wrist in a box of crackers, half-empty before you know it. And that evening you explode in an angry outburst at your spouse, blindsiding you both. You ask yourself, where did *that* come from? And if you do have an idea about the origins, is there a way to navigate these vicissitudes of life more skillfully—so they don't hobble you the rest of the day, only to overwhelm you later?

Mindfulness pulls back the veil between inner cause and outer effect, opening the door to being more present and authentically connected— with the moment, with others, and with ourselves. And just as the heavenly bodies influenced by Planet Nine are the clues leading scientists to her discovery, with mindfulness our habits of thinking and reactivity can be skillfully navigated, disentangling us from the weight of unproductive, painful patterns.

This leads to profound changes in our thought patterns and responses. It reverses obscuration of our endogenous qualities of calm, compassion, and peace. New clarity of mind and inner confidence emerge—qualities that translate directly to greater happiness, ease of living, clearer communications with others, tranquility, and freedom.

Change Your Mind—Change Your Brain

What you do with your mind shapes your brain. With mindfulness practice, you do little things with the mind that lead to big changes in your brain and your experience of living. Mindfulness is a form of mental development and a particular kind of awareness you bring to your life and daily activities that, confirmed by thousands of research studies on mindfulness and mindfulness meditation, allows you to reform reactivity while cultivating positive brain states. Through mindfulness practice, you can reform and restore your inner mental mass—your personal planet—for the better. Thanks to neuroplasticity, newly shaped neural circuits allow you to more effectively manage unsettling states of mind, emotions, stress, anxiety, and other troubling mood states, revealing your innate happiness, love, and wisdom. You discover a new freedom from being on autopilot—with everything from eating to navigating conversations.

The Mindfulness-Vegan Connection

Traditionally, mindfulness practice is supported by the three pillars of ethics, concentration, and wisdom. Ethics includes not causing unnecessary harm to others and non-greed, such as demonstrated by our food choices. This elevates our mindfulness practice by grounding us in compassion and generosity, granting us more ease of heart. Concentration trains us in steadiness of mind. Together, these lead to wisdom, which opens up the understanding of our own true nature and insights into the nature of life itself.

By aspiring to live vegan, you've already made a choice that is fundamentally ethical and mindful. It means you are already aware, watchful, careful, attentive—*mindful*—of the bigger picture: Earth's environmental predicament, the well-being of the creatures that we share her with, and your health. All simply by choosing what you put on your fork.

The Challenges

Vegan living is fast gaining momentum. The number of people veering away from animal products in favor of eating a plant-based diet is rapidly on the rise. For some people, this shift from the omnivorous norm has been initially easy. For others, transition has taken a little more time. Yet there can be hurdles beyond kitchen basics. Some of these challenges are not necessarily unfamiliar. Others are new. Based on more than 1,600 surveys submitted in preparation for this book, these challenges fall into two main areas: personal and social.

Personal

Even for those who have acquired the kitchen skills needed for vegan living, there can be stumbling blocks that can cripple desired outcomes—or derail them entirely. These problems, which can affect people of all dietary persuasions, can show up as mindless snacking, stress or emotionally reactive eating, and cravings. Lack of being prepared with good food on hand can get in the way of the best intentions. Self-imposed dietary rigidity that taints the occasional vegan "treat" with tension—or worry about "making a mistake"—can suck all the joy out of the eating experience. These undermine attempts at lasting lifestyle change. They keep personal happiness and peace—let alone the pure joy of eating and thriving at your naturally healthy weight—out of reach.

Social

When your way of eating rubs up against the animal product–laced cultural and familial status quo, there can be unexpected trials. As you reframe your nutrition to be plant exclusive, resistance from family and friends can present, well, difficulties. The stress surrounding these points of conflict can be very disheartening. This intensifies the anxiety many vegans already feel about the truths surrounding food choice: the dramatic impact of animal agriculture on environmental degradation and the avalanche of suffering caused by the inclusion of animal products in the diet.

These challenges—issues related to eating and stress points surrounding ethical considerations of food—have something fundamental
in common. They aren't about what's on the plant-based plate or how to
make a good vegan soup. These challenges are of an *inner* nature. That
means a solution of an inner nature is called for.

Enter Mindfulness

We react with automaticity in many situations throughout the day.
These reactions to the daily ups and downs of life—reactions that can
play themselves out in eating habits, interactions with other people, and
with ourselves—can be the source of a great deal of personal pain.

Mindfulness offers something new by putting in your hands tools for
effectively navigating these challenges and meeting any situation in a
more balanced way. With mindfulness practice, even in the face of difficulties, you become aware of reactivity in a unique fashion that allows
you to make more skillful choices. This gives birth to a new freedom
around food. A new ease in navigating difficult situations and conversations emerges, helping you effectively manage the reactivity that can
exaggerate philosophical differences. When you can be more fully present, you develop the capacity to respond wisely and with less reactivity
in any circumstance.

Not surprisingly, mindfulness is also a proven antidote to stress, giving us some of the deepest research surrounding its practical application. Mindfulness is being implemented by hundreds of hospitals, health
practitioners, and other similar settings due to its ability to change how
our brain responds to stress.[3]

Just about everyone who responded to the Mindful Vegan Survey
said they want an increased sense of mental and emotional equilibrium,
greater ease with managing moods and unproductive habits of reactivity,
less stress eating and mindless eating, greater clarity and confidence in
talking with friends and family about what's on their plate, and being at
greater ease with their body. Responders who already practice mindfulness or some form of meditation responded as already enjoying a higher
degree of these very qualities, relative to those who do not already have
a routine.

The Mindful Vegan—The Next Leg of Your Journey

The Mindful Vegan opens the door to creating a more resilient vegan lifestyle, liberating you from brain lock with old thinking patterns and enabling you to live more joyfully with food. It sets you on a path to finding a more balanced, peaceful life and to being a better communicator about urgent issues and lifestyle choices. It offers solutions to the dilemma that food can present in a way that is personally satisfying and aligned with your deepest values. It is for anyone who wants to be free of frustrating and baffling eating behaviors and discover their naturally healthy body and weight. It is for anyone who wants to find an antidote to the stress that comes as companion to conscious living and eating. It offers an anchor in times of confusion and transition. Mindfulness gives you the ability to see your experiences more clearly and be present with greater balance. *The Mindful Vegan* is the first book in both the mindful living and vegan realms that creates a supportive platform for and unites the two.

Though mindfulness may sound exotic, I'll take the mystery out of it. I'll show you how you can cultivate mindfulness and reap its proven benefits—without complex training or lots of spare time. First, I'll explain what mindfulness means. I'll show the many ways that it has been successfully implemented so that you can get as excited as I am about how mindfulness applies to the challenges we've described. You'll discover some of the research surrounding mindfulness, how it works, and why mindfulness-based intervention programs are being taught by psychologists, scientists, athletes, lawyers, professors, therapists—professionals from all walks of life.[4]

How to Use This Book

First, I'll detail the basics for starting a mindfulness practice. From there, lessons are presented over the course of thirty days. Day One starts with one minute of formal mindfulness meditation practice. Each day we will add another minute of practice. Thus, on Day Two you will practice for two minutes, Day Three for three minutes, and so on. This way your practice is built in a very accessible, progressive fashion. Sound simple? *Simple is the new advanced.*

You are certainly welcome to practice longer than the established time for each day. Yet commitment to practice each day is important, as the skills you build in barely noticeable increments provide greater potential for you to enjoy the benefits that mindfulness practice brings.

As you build your meditation practice through the thirty-day plan, we'll simultaneously take a deeper look at how many of the problems that are part of our life experience can be transformed with mindfulness, and how to cultivate mindful living so that you can start enjoying the benefits, just as I have. I'll teach you strategies that you can easily implement to navigate difficult mental states, decoupling the link between craving and unwanted behaviors, thus dismantling addiction loops and leading to the fading of craving itself. You'll find out how mindfulness of the body and breath is the critical first step for learning how to regulate negative thought loops and emotions. You'll also discover how a whole-food vegan plate invites you to eat in harmony with your body's hunger and fullness signals, making it the best match for realizing your naturally healthy body and weight.

Every day will include four elements, each noted with an icon for easy recognition:

formal meditation practice, the duration of which is noted at the beginning of each lesson

notation of the audio guide option

lesson for the day, including research-based benefits of mindfulness

a mindful moment, inspiration for the day

Throughout the book, you'll find quotes and personal vignettes from my own experience and those of my students, along with tips for practice, additional insights, and inspiration. You'll discover examples of how to draw upon your mindfulness practice to navigate challenges of living so that you can live with greater ease and happiness.

There is no requirement that the entire plan be completed within the thirty days. You can take as long as you like with each week. Likewise, there is no requirement that you take thirty days to complete the course if you want to move more quickly. For example, you could realistically complete Day One through Day Five on the first day if you want to dive deeper into practice right away. You can read the entire book first and then go back through day by day to support your mindfulness practice. You can jump ahead to chapter topics of keen interest, while continuing to move forward with daily lessons. The four-week format simply provides structure so that you can proceed in clear, doable fashion from day one. And if you need more time, take more time. The important thing is consistent, daily practice of mindfulness meditation, to which the benefits are dose respondent. And you can go through the course again and again, as often as you like. I'll also serve up a handful of tasty, healthy vegan recipes at the end of the book—to keep you mindful of the joy of eating wonderful, delicious, and satisfying food that brings enjoyment and ethics in harmony.

You are embarking on a journey that can deeply enrich, support, and transform your life experience. Getting started and practice from day one are key—which is why I have organized this book into daily lessons. Mindfulness is a recipe that can be applied to every facet of your life. Guided by the discoveries you make about your own inner planet, you may discover a new perspective that shifts, for the better, your relationship to life.

Audio Guides

To assist your meditation practice, I have created audio guides to accompany each of the thirty days. These can be downloaded free of charge online; for more information, see Resources (page 265). Several of these audio guides are also available on the Insight Timer app: navigate to Lani Muelrath and download selected audios for The Mindful Vegan Book Meditation Practice.

Each audio download is the same length of time as the practice time designated for each day. Thus, the audio download for Day One is one minute in length, Day Two is two minutes, and so on. The first few days, I provide guided instructions for the entire length of the audio. As the days progress, though each day's audio will open with guidance, there will be increasing segments of silence so that you can continue practice uninterrupted until the end of the recording is signaled. On some of the audios I will include short instructions incorporating the day's lesson, noted in the title of that particular day's audio guide. If you prefer to do meditation practice without the audio support, you can set a timer on your phone or timepiece to signal the finish. If you would like to practice longer or shorter than provided for any day, yet still take advantage of the guided practice, you can begin the day's practice with the provided audio and then set a timer for the amount of time you intend to practice.

PART ONE

freedom

Between stimulus and response there is a space.
In that space is the power to choose our response.
In our response lies our growth and our freedom.

—Viktor Frankl

on to something

The curious paradox is that when I accept myself just as I am, then I can change.

—CARL ROGERS

THE MINUTE I STEPPED into my pantry, I knew I was on to something big. I had entered to fetch a few ingredients for dinner. As I reached for a jar of rice, out of the corner of my eye, nestled on the shelf in familiar wrapping, there it was. A big chunk of chocolate. I had put it there some two weeks earlier. I had forgotten all about it.

Between you and me, I never forget there's chocolate in the house. Up until that moment, that is. As a (now ex-) career dieter who used to consider myself an emotional, compulsive overeater, certain I was "addicted" to sweets, chocolate in the house—or ice cream, or cookies, or anything in the dessert family—had always been a preoccupational hazard. So perhaps you can understand why forgetting that there was chocolate in the pantry was, for me, a huge sign of hope.

Why had I forgotten about the chocolate? What had changed? At that moment, I realized that a new element in my life—mindfulness practice—had opened a remarkable newfound ease in my relationship with food, eating, and my body. Forgetting about the chocolate was not a memory lapse. Rather, it flagged the dissolving of a previous obsession. I was experiencing a new freedom around food that I had thought, up to this point in time, was possible only in my dreams. And it led to my body happily settling into a naturally healthy weight—roughly fifty pounds lighter than my highest—via an entirely different pathway than I had explored before.

As a matter of fact, mindfulness superseded every other tool for change I have ever known. The usual change-your-behavior battle cries for food attitudes—regimented food plans, reward systems, amping up motivation, affirmations, removing "temptation," goal setting—were largely rendered obsolete through this one simple practice. It wasn't long before I realized that mindfulness had shifted, for the better, my relationship to just about everything else in my life, too.

Imagine

Mindfulness is a simple mental practice that can dramatically increase your innate capacity for experiencing inner happiness and peace. This fresh capacity then shows up everywhere—and that means in the eating realm, too, the first place that the effects of mindfulness were evidenced so strongly for me. For example...

- Imagine being emancipated from the grip that stress or mindless eating has on your food choices, your health, and, most of all, your peace of mind.
- Imagine enjoying each morsel of your vegan meals without an unrelenting inner dialogue that overanalyzes every bite, free of an ongoing inner warfare between what you want to eat and your "won't" power.
- Imagine the liberation of truly savoring that delicious dessert without the fear that once you start, you won't be able to stop.
- Imagine being released from the stress of an expectation of "perfection," finding yourself in a new dimension of ease in your body, and discovering your naturally healthy weight.

Further . . .

- Imagine navigating conversations with others about eating—and living—vegan, with greater clarity, equanimity, and presence of mind.

- Imagine being more grounded in the joy, compassion, ethics, vision, and integrity of vegan living, so you can steer your way more confidently through the sometimes rocky seas of modern life and the current culinary culture.
- Imagine sustaining an inner connectivity and resiliency, helping you thrive as an ambassador for conscious living.

Sound like the kind of ease you'd like to experience more of? I now enjoy these freedoms more each day. Mindfulness has been the linchpin for me. Mindfulness has also made the difference for thousands of others. Using what we now know about the capabilities of the mind, mindfulness can be an answer for living with greater ease for you, too.

What's the Canary in *Your* Coal Mine?

In this chapter, I'll tell you more about mindfulness and how it can operate as an antidote to what troubles you. I'll show you how it can revolutionize your relationship with food and your body, should this be something you seek. If eating issues are the canary in your coal mine, trying to control the problem with a rigid diet, self-confrontation, or distracting yourself—even chewing each bite fifty times—doesn't get to the heart of the matter. Here, and throughout this book, I'll share with you how practicing mindfulness brings freedom and a new joy to your eating experience.

What if issues in the eating realm aren't your personal waterloo? No matter what your point of pain, mindfulness can help you navigate life's difficulties. We all differ in our reactivity to disquieting states. Some people cope by staying chronically overbusy. Others turn anxiety and unsettled emotion into a driving exercise schedule. Some deal with life's discomforts by being obsessed with productivity or perfectionism, becoming workaholics, aspiring to acquire more things or accomplishments, or succumbing to other distractive or addictive behaviors. Perhaps cravings—for food, for recognition, for checking your email or Instagram feed—have become a preoccupation. Some get locked into a hyperstressed state, thinking they need it to get things done—yet finding that they are simply achieving, for the most part, chronic stress and anxiety.

Mindfulness practice reaches beyond your plate to positively impact every aspect of your life. It goes under the surface of that which troubles you, giving you a simple solution for many of life's ups and downs by revolutionizing and rewiring your reactivity to them, thus shifting your inner landscape. Let's look at some of the documented benefits of mindfulness, underscored by the research, and how they can play out on your plate.

Mindfulness and Freedom

In the past decade, several studies have assessed alterations in the brain related to mindfulness. Multiple measurements show correlations between brain changes and mindfulness meditation practice, reflected in stress reduction, emotion regulation, and increased well-being.[1]

How might this play out for you, personally? Among other benefits, it has been demonstrated that with mindfulness, you can:

- Increase self-awareness of and lessen harmful patterns of feeling, thought, and reactivity[2]
- Enhance positive emotions, self-confidence, well-being, patience, and compassion[3]
- Experience more calm in the midst of a hectic life, creating a greater capacity to deal with adverse events and situations[4]
- Reduce stress, anxiety, and depression, and improve moods[5]
- Quiet your mind from intrusive, energy-sapping thoughts[6]
- Increase mental clarity and focus, improve working memory, and tame your wandering mind[7]
- Enhance creativity and improve insightful problem-solving[8]
- Reduce relapses in substance use disorders[9]
- Improve immune function[10]
- Enjoy a happier, more positive outlook[11]
- Improve cognitive function, mental stamina, and resilience[12]
- Reduce insomnia and better manage pain[13]

Mindfulness-based instruction has also become a hot research topic in the progression of Alzheimer's disease from mild cognitive impairment, due to the positive impact of mindfulness-based instruction on adverse factors such as stress, depression, and metabolic syndrome as risk factors in neurodegeneration.[14] How can one simple practice impact this breadth of scenarios, making shifts as fundamental as these possible? How can the same thing that gets us out of a troubled relationship with food ease your way with life's other challenges?

Emerging research on mindfulness might make it seem like a cure-all for life's problems. Living mindfully does not, however, hand you a trouble-free world. Rather, it provides a pathway for you to live a full and contented life in a world in which both joys and challenges are a given by opening your awareness of and changing your relationship with the present.[15]

We are used to our thoughts wandering in free-form fashion, often leading us willy-nilly into long-established patterns of reactivity. Mindfulness is a mechanism that brings what are otherwise unconscious behavior patterns to conscious awareness where you can do something about them—somewhat like disarming land mines instead of detonating them. Mindfulness opens a space of awareness around your urges and reactions. It gives you a virtual foot in the door, expanding that moment between stimulus and reactivity. You gain new access to the choice of where to place your attention, rather than having your attention taken hostage by reactive thoughts and emotions.

Once you open the door to the possibilities of choice, you can more freely choose your responses.[16] By practicing the conscious directing of your attention in the present moment, you open up the space to living more consciously. You disentangle yourself from problematic habits, beliefs, and conditioning, so you can make more skillful choices in every area of your life. You give yourself back the full power of choice—and with it, ultimate freedom. This is authentic, from-the-inside change.

The Mindfulness, Food, and Eating Connection

As you *live* more mindfully, you *eat* more mindfully. Rather than being shackled to an eating regimen—trying to muscle a change from the outside and hoping it will "take"—mindfulness teaches you to skillfully navigate the complexities of what, when, and how much you eat, no matter what the circumstances.[17]

As a practicing or aspiring vegan, you are probably already mindful of the many ways that your food choices impact your health, our planet Earth, and the other beings with whom we share her. Regular mindfulness practice multiplies, deepens, and broadens these benefits, leading to significant life improvements.[18] Here are some specific ways mindfulness has been shown to fundamentally improve a relationship with food and overcome behaviors that contribute to health challenges:

- Dismantle destructive eating habits such as mindless eating[19]
- Dissolve compulsive or addictive behavior patterns[20]
- Decrease chronic stress, emotional eating, and stress-related hormone production, which leads to deposit of abdominal fat, contributing to metabolic syndrome[21]
- Dramatically reduce and eliminate binge eating[22]
- Restore the pure joy of eating and release the struggle, negative self-judgment, and inner conflict often associated with eating in any setting[23–24]
- Reconnect you with your natural hunger and fullness signals—and your naturally healthy weight[25]

Sounds (even in part) like your wish list? The tally goes on, but let's take a closer look at how mindfulness can lead to significant changes in your relationship with food and why. This provides us with a good model for the change you may be seeking in any domain of behavior in which you experience stress or reactivity.

The New Frontier

In contrast to diet books filled with rules and charts, you will find something completely new in *The Mindful Vegan*. In fact, you might no longer look at standard methods of dietary regimentation in quite the same way. They are eclipsed by what mindfulness quite literally brings to the table. With mindfulness, by getting to the heart of the problem, you disentangle the struggles often associated with food.

The Mindful Vegan will show you how to rewire your personal relationship with food and eating and forge a new one of ease, peace, and freedom. You will discover a new inner connection that truly satisfies, deepening the pleasure and peace that come with eating in alignment with your ethical ideals. You will find out how to move from habits of reactivity to responding in ways that put you in charge of what you eat. You become more confident, comfortable, relaxed, and free to simply enjoy food and experience greater ease with making health-building choices. You become reconnected with your natural hunger and fullness signals that have become obscured by a busy mind, a busy life, a regimented food plan—or all three. Mindfulness gets to the roots of your challenges around food—whether it's refurbishing old habits, employing self-regulation of emotions, or becoming more at ease and grounded in vegan living. Mindfulness can be the deciding factor between successful adoption of a healthy vegan diet or repeated frustrated attempts.

Through mindfulness of emotions, thoughts, and bodily sensations, you gain tools for being in the presence of conflict in a kind, compassionate way. As you undertake this training, you learn to let the mind settle so that insight into right action can arise—an indispensable aid to navigating conversations and other situations. An equanimity emerges, helping you move from reactivity to more skillful response. You still work hard for what you care about and take action accordingly. Yet you cultivate a dimension of compassion and understanding. Instead of approaching change through antagonism and anger, you embody the qualities of the cause through cultivating steadiness and a good heart.

Mindfulness Demystified

Mindfulness is commonly described as consciously attending to your moment-to-moment experience. This awakens us to our habits of thinking and our mental conditioning. We become willing and able to take a step back from our usual autopilot and reactivity, the conditions in which we go through many of our days—unless we cultivate the practice of doing otherwise.

Ordinarily, our attention swings rather wildly. Our thoughts carry us all over the place via random thoughts, fleeting memories, enchanting fantasies, or tidbits of something we've seen or heard—right down to the ubiquitous ad jingle. Mindfulness meditation is used to develop the skill, or state, of mindfulness. This practice diminishes distraction through sustained attention to the movements of the mind itself. Rather than being swept away and captured by a thought, feeling, or emotion, with mindfulness meditation you gently observe your thoughts and feelings as they come and go. It is through this process that the qualities of being more mindful emerge.

Two Aspects of Mindfulness

Mindfulness has been described as the opposite of automaticity. As awareness with a quality of attentiveness, mindfulness training strengthens your "attentional muscles" so that you can more skillfully direct your attention. The awareness that emerges is a by-product of cultivating the following two components—the combination of which is unique to mindfulness training.[26]

1 **Self-Regulation of Your Attention**
   First, you train your mind to focus through the use of a particular phenomenon, such as the feeling of the breath. This results in an increased awareness of events as they unfold—in your thoughts and emotions, in your body, and in the world around you. You start to notice your habits of reactivity to these events. By steadying your awareness on your immediate experience, you learn to let go of thoughts and feelings that distract you from the present moment and pull you into ruminations about the past—or worries about the future. Such distractedness breeds confusion, anxiety, stress, and emotional turmoil.

2. **Orientation to Your Experience**
   The second aspect of mindfulness training involves keeping an attitude of kindness, patience, and acceptance about where the mind wanders whenever it drifts away from the breath or other center of focus, as it inevitably will. You cultivate equanimity toward thoughts, feelings, and sensations that arise. By acknowledging and observing them, you create a stance of acceptance that opens you to the possibilities of the present moment.

Together, with these two aspects of mindfulness practice, you culti-vate your capacity not only to see things just as they are from moment to moment but also to be present with them with greater ease.[27] The ability to sustain your attentive awareness—mindfully, with curiosity and calmness—brings greater clarity and insight. This allows you to acknowledge many activities of your mind without getting caught up with them. Through this process, you unearth the ability to make more skillful choices of thought, word, and deed. This ability to choose is what makes change possible.[28]

Doing vs. Being

In contrast to the modern habit and cultural urge to go, do, have, acquire, produce, distract, and otherwise stay busy, mindfulness invites you to breathe and be in the present. You learn to use your attention to shift between a *doing* mode of mind and a *being* mode of mind as needed. Striving, perceiving thoughts as facts, avoiding unpleasant experiences, and brooding over future events are all aspects of a "doing" mode of mind. In contrast, "being" is characterized by having conscious awareness of the point where reactions begin, seeing thoughts as mental events, and remaining in the present moment. The ability to recognize these modes of your mind and developing the skill to shift between them opens up choices. Being aware of the mind's tendencies and habits strengthens your ability to choose how to respond in the moment—the only time you can really make a different choice. In these choices lies your freedom.[29]

Most people find the notion of meditation—the idea of discovering how to simply "be"—highly appealing. Intuitively we respond to the idea somewhat like a thirsty person to the sound of a distant stream. Yet nothing in our culture or schooling has taught us how to steady our attention in order to be in this stillness. By cultivating mindfulness, you learn how to shift into "being" mode. Growing this awareness extends the ability we all already have to know what is actually happening, as it is happening, in the mind itself, including thoughts, feelings, and reactivity. You become engaged in a way that helps you let go of trou-bling thoughts and behaviors. By giving you specific tools of acknowl-edging and being present with your feelings and thoughts—including unsettling tension and anxiety—mindfulness assists you in living more skillfully with all of life's ups and downs.

As you learn to be present with thoughts, emotions, and physical responses as they arise, you disarm the potential they have to overwhelm you. Rather than having them continue to drive you to diffuse anxiety and tension through reactivity, mindless eating, short-tempered outbursts, or any other way you have of playing out stress, you restore the freedom to make more skillful choices.

Autopilot Antidote

Ever find yourself stuck in negative thinking loops? Are you ever hopelessly caught up in eating (or other) habits that not only aren't helping you but are keeping you ensnared in a frustrating frame of mind? If you're not in the present moment, then where the heck are you? And why does it matter?

We are, most of the time, operating on autopilot: driving, eating, even talking—we're lost in thought, rehashing the past or rehearsing for the future, missing life as it unfolds. Mindfulness brings something new to the table—conscious awareness.

Through mindfulness, you develop a remarkable ability to navigate troubling thoughts and habitual behavior. You learn to cultivate openness, curiosity, and willingness to be with what is in the present moment rather than play out your old patterns of thinking and reactivity.

As you interrupt negative aspects of being on autopilot, can you see how this might dismantle old patterns that are holding you back? With this kind of mindful presence you discover a new enjoyment of eating and ease around food and your body. With interpersonal relationships, you become aware of patterns of reactivity that cause inner turmoil and get in the way of effective communication. You open the door to bringing more equanimity to each interaction.

By giving you the power to self-regulate emotions and direct your thoughts in a compassionate, friendly fashion, mindfulness helps you replace mindless, compulsive behavior with fresh, positive responses.[30] This opens the door to liberation from negative patterns—bringing with it an unprecedented inner sense of freedom and peace.

The Chocolate Connection

My chocolate-in-the-pantry incident is a clear, real-life application and result of mindfulness training and practice. First, diminished accumulation of emotional reactivity, a modified stress response, greater calm and reduced anxiety—direct outcomes of mindfulness practice—had directly and positively impacted my well-being. Instead of being constantly mired in my thoughts, building a wall of tension and anxiety around eating and the greater specter of life's challenges, mindfulness gave me practice in being present with emotions, thoughts, and feelings in a more conscious way. This in turn disassembled a long-held pattern of reactivity to accumulated stress and unsettled states. Striking at the root of my problems around food and eating, the habit of reaching for food in reactivity was neutralized, which resulted in direct positive impact on personal happiness in the eating arena—and beyond. Second, my mental habit of being preoccupied with certain foods in the environment was transformed. By creating that "space" between stimulus and response, I had learned how to manage thoughts or urges—for example, a draw to chocolate in the house—in a way that allowed me to live more skillfully.

I wanted to live more freely and joyfully around food, not spend my time strategizing how to hide from chocolate. Mindfulness delivered this in a way no other "program" had approached before. It is what allowed me to give up dieting for good and mindfully turn to my natural hunger and fullness signals instead. It is what made it possible for me to open up to the pure enjoyment of eating, shed a fair amount of poundage and the inner discomfort surrounding it, and sustain these changes for decades.

I suspect that you are already thinking of how mindfulness might liberate your eating experience and social situations, and the endless ways that mindfulness can be of benefit to your life. As you become more skilled in mindfulness, you start to become aware of the tremendous possibility of each moment.

In the end, mindfulness is something that needs to be practiced and experienced in order to really be understood. But don't take my word for it. One of the cornerstones of mindfulness practice is realizing the benefits for yourself. No time like the present.

my watershed moment

When one thought ends, right before the next thought begins, there is a tiny gap called "now." Over time we learn to expand that gap.

—SPRING WASHAM, meditation teacher

IT IS A MOMENT I'll never forget.

As I sat down to the midday meal, I was blindsided by a tightening in my chest, followed by a squeeze in my throat. I felt as if I could barely breathe. Accompanied by a knot in my stomach the size of Manhattan, I knew something monumental was taking place.

No, I wasn't having a heart attack. But the impact of this event was no less far-reaching. For it was at this moment that a pivotal change took place in my life. It led to liberating me from a painful, troubled relationship with food. A relationship that had played itself out over decades of unsettled eating patterns, a tiresome preoccupation with dieting, constant self-criticism of my body, and the heartache of yo-yoing weight.

This moment heralded a dramatic new freedom, happiness, and peace with food that I celebrate to this day. Restoring the pure joy of eating, it ushered in an era of ease with food and my body that has proliferated into greater well-being in every area of my life. All of these shifts I can trace directly back to that instant nearly twenty-five years ago.

One thing leveraged this dramatic change in my life: mindfulness meditation practice.

My Mindful Journey

More than forty years ago, along with teaching yoga and adopting a vegetarian diet, I began a meditation practice. It wasn't the mindfulness meditation practice I am sharing with you in this book. It was a different technique. Though my aspirations were all seventies spiritual, between you and me, I was looking for a solution to my food and weight problem, and I had hoped that meditation would do it.

I gave this technique my all, even traveling to remote regions of India several times. I would get up at three in the morning to sit for hours in meditation every day. Though I did learn how to sit still for long periods of time, and cultivated a bit of concentration, these practices never made a detectable dent in my food problem. As a matter of fact, I returned from one of those trips to India noticeably pudgier than when I left from pounding down handfuls of the roasted cashews, glucose biscuits, and endless buttery curries served at the ashram.

About ten years later, browsing through a bookstore while traveling, I came across a small book about mindfulness meditation. It explained how this practice—also known as *Vipassana*, or Insight, Meditation— could give us insight into our thoughts and emotions, help us simply be present with our feelings instead of trying to figure them out or escape them, and open up our capacity for equanimity.* I was immediately interested. Instinctively, I felt this might get to the root of my food problem. The book didn't, however, include any how-to instructions. And I couldn't find anything more about it. There were far fewer resources available at the time. The internet was still in the toddler stage, Amazon wasn't born yet, and research was conducted via library card.

Returning home, I kept the book close and simultaneously dove right into completing my master's degree and launching my TV show. Meanwhile, I continued to ponder why—though happily married, with gainful employment and a promising career blooming—I couldn't seem

---

* *Vipassana* means seeing realistically. Nonsectarian and not affiliated with any ethnic or political group, with no religious or philosophical trappings, it is differentiated from other ancient forms of meditation by the fact that it is approachable by everyone. Paul R. Fleischman, MD, *An Ancient Path* (Onalaska, WA: Vipassana Research Publications, 2008), p. 13.

to get a grip on this one area of my life: food and eating. My devotion to the meditation practice I had been doing gradually waned.

I dabbled in diets for another ten years, yet I kept circling back to the mindfulness book. Finally, I decided it was time to see if the benefits it seemed to offer were for me. I signed up for a retreat to learn mindfulness meditation. Located in the foothills of Yosemite National Park, it was a ten-day silent retreat.

That's right. Silent. The purpose of the silence is to keep all outer distractions to a minimum. Just you and your body, thoughts, and emotions. Silence is where the curious gymnastics of our minds—from elaborate stories we spawn around our experiences to obsessive thinking loops to our particular avenues of escape from the vicissitudes of life, a constant parade of inner distractions—come into full view. Silence allows us to dive into this interior landscape—in a way that our usual day-to-day lives don't. Mindfulness, together with willingness, kindness, and patience, allows us to be present with all of it in a way that directly defuses our troubles.

I took to the silence like a fish to water. It was actually great respite not to have to activate one's personality with the usual social interactions. Yet as much as I relished the time "alone," navigating my inner landscape brought its own set of challenges.

Watershed Moment

It was on day four of the retreat that the episode I opened this chapter with took place. I had just sat down to the midday meal, to be eaten in silence in keeping with retreat tradition, when I was overwhelmed by the experience that I described. One of the techniques of mindfulness practice is to be willing to look at physical sensations as they arise in the body—curiously, and without judgment or avoidance. So I turned my attention to the chest squeeze, the tightness in my throat, just to observe them for what they might have to teach me.

Immediately, I was flooded with insight. I realized how much tension and anxiety I had around food and eating. And I realized that I had probably been having this experience for years. I had exacerbated it with every new diet and underscored it with every feeling of guilt or other bad feelings about food, with each moment of admonition about eating and shame about my weight.

These emotions, I realized, had been there for a long, long time. I just hadn't been aware of them. Instead, I had been playing out stress with another batch of cookie dough or preoccupation about the next diet. Inner discomforts had, for me, rallied into what had become an obsession—for when I wasn't fixated on how I might conjure up a more dramatic weight-loss project, I was getting caught up in food cravings. Mindfulness practice was now giving me specific tools with which to address all of it. This insightful moment had two predominant qualities. I felt sorrow as I thought how sad it was that I had been having this experience for so many years—decades even. At the same time, it was a light-filled, expansive moment because of the insight I experienced around my food and eating problem.

Instantly, I felt a great flood of compassion for myself. Instead of living on autopilot and reactivity with my discomforts, I simply started choosing more and more often to be *willing* to be with what was present in the moment. This experience officially opened the world of mindfulness to me. It gave me firsthand experience of the transformation that can be experienced by being fully present and how the experience can change someone in an instant. Once you know, you can't not. Looking back, the more I learn about myself, the more I believe I was probably feeling those tensions and anxieties much of the time, even outside of mealtimes. I simply never had the courage—even more, the basic tools—to realize and face them. All this time, I'd been thinking it was all about the food. But that was just part of the problem. Eating just happened to be the highly charged water I was swimming in at the moment the insight came.

I began to see past the promise of the cookie dough—or whatever form it might take on any particular day. Not out of punitiveness, or with willpower, but out of realizing that the sanctuary I sought in food was false, empty. With mindfulness practice I began to see past this agent of transitory asylum to the pain and confusion that always followed. This came as a natural outgrowth, organically emerging from the mindful experience. Looking clearly at our mental and emotional landscape, along with the physical sensations that are part of our moment-to-moment experience, reveals more to us about our experience than we can imagine. It is really quite remarkable that something so simple as being mindfully present with these phenomena can have such profound effect on our ability to find our way through obstacles that are so often hidden from view.

Decision

In that moment of insight at the retreat, I realized that focusing on the food was simply skirting the issue. I made the decision to abandon dieting altogether and travel the path of mindfulness. If the door to navigating this longtime obstacle could be so immediately unlocked and opened, what else might I discover that would illuminate the pathway and lighten my load, if I were willing to investigate?

From that point on, things between me and food changed. I stopped thinking of myself as some kind of food addict or compulsive eater. I stopped repeatedly trying to eat less to shed some pounds, in favor of reconnecting with my hunger and fullness signals—the connection with which is essential to eating mindfully. Chronically cutting back muddies our true hunger and fullness indicators, causes overeating, and is the single biggest driving factor behind food blowouts and binges. Previously, I could overeat with the best of them. But I never again had one binge incident.

While I worked briefly with a coach to help me navigate the uncertainty of letting go of dieting as I knew it, it is the tools of mindfulness meditation practice that walked me through the enormous wall of fear that letting go of these controls around food, eating, and weight presented, and opened the door to unprecedented freedom. Micromanaging and analyzing every bite and obsessing over body weight and size mask underlying stress, anxiety, and not-good-enough syndrome. And heaven knows it's reinforced by our culture and cemented by the diet industry. It's one thing to read about these problems and associations and an entirely different thing to steer right through the middle of the unsettling mess. The discomforts of the loss of the familiar, even though the familiar may be painful, can be disquieting as you let go of outmoded illusions of control and move into new, uncharted territory. Without a way to navigate the seas, you continue to spin in the whirlpool.

As I continued to practice mindfulness meditation, moments of quiet, glimpses into a peaceful mind, and the growing ability to let go of the grip of obsessive thinking edified my practice. Obsessive thinking of any kind is a place we seek refuge from our restlessness and fears. We might feel anxious and seek refuge in food, other substances, or surfing the internet. We might feel insecure and seek refuge in a relentless drive for recognition or monetary success. We might feel shame and obsessively enslave ourselves to the pursuit of body perfection. Yet all false refuges respond to an interested and caring attention. We can listen to the energies behind our obsessive thinking, respond to what needs attention, and spend less and less time removed from the presence that nurtures our lives. We experience more and more often the freeing qualities of simply being present.

Over the years, my relationship to food moved in a couple of directions. For one, as I became more consciously connected with the problems perpetuated by dairy—the last vestiges of animal products in my diet—I moved from vegetarian to vegan. For several years, on the way to the school where I taught, I would drive through rolling green hills in which dairy cows grazed. As I passed them, I would sink down in my car seat with apologies in my heart and on my lips. "I'm sorry!" I would whisper. Off and on inspired to make the switch to vegan, I would come and go from eating yogurt and cheese. The awareness of inner dissonance grew with my mindfulness practice. Finally, one day, realization of the unsettling inner state I was perpetuating pushed dairy off my plate. What a difference in lightness of heart and integrity the driving-to-work experience became.

I remain watchful and alert to the many faces that obsessions around food and eating can present. I constantly see them play themselves out in people who come to me for help with their weight, food, and eating problems. Often it shows up as anxiety channeled into micromanagement of even the healthiest of foods. Overanalyzing and replaying one plant-based food plan after another, conflicted about the one right answer—they are unaware that, a large part of the time, the obsession itself is holding them back. We deal with our disquieting states and worries by hiding behind the skirts of one preoccupation or another— or one *after* another.

With mindfulness, you are cultivating a state of being that allows all the gifts of mindfulness to unfold in your experience. You don't seek peace of mind; you create the conditions in which peace of mind can take place. You don't seek to be free of mindless eating; you foster a state of mindfulness that sheds mindless eating like a snake sheds a skin. Rather than seeking just the right thing to say, you restore equanimity, compassion, and heart, bringing a kinder, clearer presence to each conversation and encounter.

PART TWO

the thirty-day plan

In truth we are always present; we only imagine ourselves to be in one place or another.

—HOWARD COHN, Insight Meditation Teacher

presence of mind

Presence is not some exotic state that we need to search for or manufacture. In the simplest terms, it is the felt sense of wakefulness, openness, and tenderness that arise when we are fully here and now with our experience.

—TARA BRACH, *True Refuge*

E'VE ALL SAID IT.
"At least I had the presence of mind to..." or "If only I'd had the presence of mind to..."

And we all know what *presence of mind* means. It's the mental clarity to make wise choices in the moment. We simply become more mindful in the minute when it matters, opening a pathway to a more skillful response and a happier outcome.

What if every eating experience could be like that, too? What if you could easily assemble your better judgment at each meal so that you can savor every bite—without the weight of inner conflict, overanalysis, or a disheartening side dish of mealtime tension?

What if you could have more presence of mind in each conversation about vegan living and about what's on your plate? Would it help you if you could bring more heart, equanimity, and compassion to them—and every other life situation? Mindfulness cultivates your natural capacity for this kind of presence. In this chapter you will learn the simple basics of mindfulness practice. This will give you all the preparation you need for getting started on Day One.

Mindfulness: Practicing Presence of Mind

How do you know if you are "present" or not? And how do you learn how to be more so, so that you can reap the remarkable benefits of mindfulness?

"Mindfulness," says Jon Kabat-Zinn, executive director of the UMass Medical School Center for Mindfulness in Medicine, Health Care, and Society, "can be thought of as moment-to-moment awareness, cultivated by paying attention in a specific way, as non-reactively, as non-judgmentally, and as open-heartedly as possible."[1]

"Paying attention in a specific way" means through conscious direction of your awareness. I will provide you with the instructions for how to do this throughout this book.

The purpose of mindfulness practice is to grow your ability to deal with all the ups and downs of life in a more balanced way. Becoming conscious of the mental habits that shape your behavior is the first step to changing them. You learn to do this by observing, with equanimity, whatever is arising. With this equanimity, you can break habits of blind reaction and instead choose better courses of action in any situation.

As you learn to watch the functioning of your own mind in a calm and curious manner, you gain insights into your own behavior. You get to know yourself with greater clarity. You become more attuned to your emotional shifts and how to more easily manage them. You learn to disentangle yourself from your thought processes and step out of your own way. You acquire the tools with which to shift mental habits and behaviors so they serve you better.

Formal and Informal Practice

Mindfulness practice takes place in two ways: *formal* practice and *informal* practice, with the idea of developing a seamlessness between them.

Formal practice is developing mindfulness specifically through mindfulness meditation, often called sitting practice. A formal meditation can take just a couple of minutes, or it can last ten, twenty, thirty minutes, or more.

Informal practice refers to being mindfully present as much as possible during the day, no matter what you are doing—whether washing the dishes, giving a presentation at work, or walking the dog. You practice informally when you apply attentive awareness to something you are engaged in, while including in your field of vision the thoughts, emotions, and bodily sensations that arise within the situation. For instance, when eating, you attend to the sight, smell, taste, satisfaction, and enjoyment of the eating experience—including awareness of hunger and fullness as you eat and thoughts and feelings that arise. By living more mindfully with more awareness throughout the day in this fashion, you disentangle automaticity and open to the ease and happiness that comes with more present living.

Informal practice is built upon a foundation of formal practice. You wouldn't sit down to play piano in concert at Carnegie Hall without practicing piano or run an eight-hundred-meter race without practicing running. With mindfulness meditation you are practicing using your attention in a way that awakens you from—and allows you to move beyond—your ingrained habits of reaction. Your formal mindfulness practice then spills over into every aspect of your waking life in a natural way.

For both formal and informal practice, the basic instructions are the same: 1) become aware of the present-moment experience, and 2) gently redirect your attention from wandering to the present-moment experience, with kindness and patience. Actually, returning to the moment takes place as soon as you notice you've wandered off. Mindfulness is easy. It's noticing that you've wandered from it that is the challenge.

How to Establish a Daily Mindfulness Meditation Practice

Here are the basic guidelines of when, where, time, and setup instructions that will help you get started with your formal practice.

When to Practice

It is helpful to establish a regular time for your formal practice. For many people the morning is the best. Your mind may be calmer yet more energized earlier in the day than later. Also, because it is so easy for time to get away from us, if you haven't put in some time for practice early in the day, before you know it the day is gone, and along with it your opportunity for practice. Some people prefer to practice at the end of the day. Some do both. The best time to practice is that which you can realistically commit to on a regular basis. You can also break up formal practice into two or more shorter segments throughout the day. When you sit in formal practice daily, you will more quickly experience noticeable benefits such as less reactivity and stress, greater calm, and greater mindfulness around your daily activities.

Where to Practice

Your formal practice can take place anywhere—you don't need a special room. At the same time, it can be helpful to have a corner, chair, or area designated for your practice, as simply arriving at the spot helps you become more focused. But I have meditated everywhere—in airplanes, in a berth on a boat, and in airport lounges. And so can you.

Time for Practice

You may feel that you are so busy that the thought of adding one more thing to your to-do list—no matter how beneficial—seems like too much. After all, our modern lives are pulled in so many directions that busy and busier seem to be the norm. I invite you to see mindfulness practice as a simple tool for enhancing your quality of life, rather than one more thing to do. In truth, it is a way of *being* rather than *doing* and it can be suited to different lifestyles and needs. While formal practice, as I will show you, is important, mindfulness is also to be practiced as part of our everyday routine—doing the laundry, driving to work, or waiting in line at the market.

As you begin, you can start with just one minute and add more as your practice develops, which is how I have laid it out for you in this book. The typical chosen time for formal practice is between ten and forty-five minutes. Yet regardless of the time you choose, regularity of practice is key. Always keep in mind that any amount of time in practice is better than none. Any amount of time you can engage in practice is beneficial. As you experience the inner sense of ease and balance that practice develops, chances are you will want to increase practice time.

Mindfulness Meditation Setup Instructions

Once you've established a place and time for your practice, the next step is actual practice.

Remember PAIR

PAIR is a simple four-step method for gathering your attention every time you practice mindfulness meditation. PAIR stands for position, anchor, intention, and remindfulness (remember, return, repeat).

Together, we will build the practice of using these steps in the lessons ahead, starting on Day One. I describe them for you here so that you can see how they will help you get started each time you practice, and so that you can select your preferred position for Day One.

Position

You may be under the impression that sitting on a cushion on the floor is a requirement for mindfulness meditation. This may be because in many of the cultures from which the practice of mindfulness is derived, people sit on the floor more often than they sit on chairs. There are actually several positions from which to choose for formal practice: seated on a chair, seated on a cushion on the floor, sitting on your knees (with a cushion or low bench), and even lying down. I employ each of them, depending on the occasion.

If sitting cross-legged is comfortable to you, start there. If you prefer sitting in a chair to sitting on the floor, that's fine, too. The best position for formal practice is the one that will allow you to be most comfortable yet attentive for the duration of your practice. And you can always rotate positions from one sitting to another as desired. Here are more instructions to help you select your posture for formal practice.

Sitting on a floor cushion: Seat yourself tailor fashion, or any way that suits you, on a cushion on the floor. Some people discover that one advantage of the floor cushion option is that it helps you stay more attentive. You can easily situate cushions so that you create a comfortable, supportive position for practice. You should be seated slightly toward the front of the cushion so that it raises your hips a little higher than your knees, allowing your knees to drop as close as possible to the floor when you cross your legs. This eases circulation through hips and knees. It also exerts a gentle forward tilt of the pelvis that provides a solid foundation for spinal alignment. A *zafu* is a cushion designed specifically for this purpose, available online and at specialty outlets. For years I simply used an assortment of pillows from around the house, and so can you. Yet once I had a chance to try a zafu, I finally understood what all the excitement was about. You can also put cushions under one or both knees to establish comfort as needed.

Place either your pillow or zafu atop a soft mat to cushion your ankles, and you're all set. Again, your spine should be erect yet without strain. Elegant yet relaxed.

Sitting in a chair: If you choose the chair position, sit in a chair that is fairly firm yet comfortable. Now is not the time for the La-Z-Boy recliner. With your feet flat on the floor, your spine should be relaxed yet upright. If your feet do not reach the floor, place a pillow or cushion beneath them so that your knees do not drop at a steep angle from your hips. Should you need a small pillow at your lower back for support, that's fine, too. Let your hands be in a comfortable position resting on the tops of your thighs, on the arms of the chair, or folded in your lap. Your position should be one in which you feel attentive yet at ease.

Kneeling: Seat yourself on a low bench or cushion(s) placed directly beneath your buttocks. Your feet are tucked beneath the low bench or folded to the side of the cushions. Your weight should rest into the bench or cushions rather than into your knees.

Whether seated in a chair, or on the floor, or kneeling, avoid dropping into a slumped position, which can decrease concentration and generate discomfort in your back. At the same time, you may notice that it may take a while for the muscles in your back to become accustomed to what is actually excellent posture. As the small stabilizing muscles in your back quickly adapt, this will become easier.

Lying down: If for some reason you are unable to sit, you can lie on your back with your arms comfortably resting at your sides or on the front of your body. One drawback of lying down for meditation is that it can make it easier for you to slip into sleep. Yet if you have an injury or other situation that makes it difficult for you to sit in an upright position, this is a viable option. It is also convenient for getting in more practice first thing in the morning. I have found that sleep rarely overcomes me in lying down meditation, but that is after several years of practice. At the same time, I find I am more attentive when seated.

Whichever position you choose, simply be at ease and let your eyes gently close.

Anchor

Direct your awareness to the feel of your breathing at the point where it enters your body, just beneath the nose and above the upper lip. We will dive more deeply into breath as anchor on Day Two. As we progress through the thirty-day plan, we will include other anchors for practice, such as bodily sensations and emotions.

Intention

Set your intention to continue your mindfulness meditation for a specific amount of time. Deciding the duration in advance helps offset time negotiations during practice, should your mind become restless. A clock or timer is all you need. Another very important element of intention is to bring an attitude of kindness, curiosity, relaxation, equanimity, and patience to your practice.

Remindfulness

Your attention will likely wander, perhaps even before you start. As soon as you notice your mind has wandered (*remembering*), it means that mindfulness has *returned*. Bring your attention back to anchor. *Repeat.*

In Days One, Two, and Three, we'll walk through the process of establishing mindful awareness for your formal practice using PAIR. Before then, explore the different positions for formal practice and decide which you will use for Day One. You can always try a different position down the road.

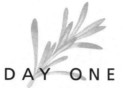

DAY ONE

beginning practice: position

Ultimately, I see mindfulness as a love affair—with life, with reality and imagination, with the beauty of your own being, with your heart and body and mind—and with the world.

—Jon Kabat-Zinn

MEDITATION PRACTICE: *1 minute*

Note: *Before today's practice, review the instructions for practice positions as described on pages 37–39. Try them out and select which is best for you.*

Day One, *Position*

The four steps of PAIR—position, anchor, intention, and remindfulness—help you gather your attention each time you sit for formal practice. Because of the structure they provide, giving purposeful attention to PAIR at first forms a solid foundation for the next thirty days and beyond. For this reason, we will devote today's practice to simply becoming more familiar with the first step in PAIR: position.

Laying the Foundation of Your Practice

Position

Move into whichever position you have chosen. Whether in a chair or on a floor cushion, your body should be upright yet relaxed. This combination keeps you comfortable and alert at the same time. You want to be attentive, yet at ease. Rest your hands wherever it is comfortable for you—on the tops of your thighs, folded in your lap, or on the arms of the chair, if a chair is your choice. If sitting is not an option for you, you can be lying down. Gently close your eyes.

To help you mentally arrive, begin by noticing your body and how it feels to be seated on the chair or cushion—right here, right now. Become aware of the touch of your feet where they meet the floor, your hips where they contact the surface beneath you. Through this process, you are bringing your mind into your body and into the present moment. Your body is always in the present moment. Your body can help you bring your mind to the present, too, just by your bringing your attention to your body.

Mentally, notice your hands. Can you feel if your hands are tense or tight? Allow them to soften. What about your arms and shoulders? Notice what they feel like right now, and let them relax by letting your shoulders drop away from the ears, while still keeping an upright posture. Let your jaw drop loose. Soften your facial muscles, letting your face become free of tension. This alone will have a dramatic effect on relaxing your entire system.

To help release any unease or strain that you may have brought with you to the moment, and to help gather your attention, take two or three deep breaths. With each exhalation, consciously let go and relax. Intentionally surrendering bodily tension will help you be more present with whatever arises during your meditation practice.

What's Your Why?

As formal instruction gets under way, reflect briefly on why you are interested in mindfulness practice. Perhaps you are drawn to experience some of the proven benefits listed in part one. Maybe you recognize in yourself some of the difficulties presented by reactivity or a wandering mind. It may be that you are seeking relief from detractors from your daily experience—agitation, anxiety, impatience, mental distraction, or other unsettled states that play themselves out in negative moods, mindless eating, or frustrating reactivity.

It can be helpful to bring to mind at the start of each meditation practice period—sometimes referred to as "sitting"—what has inspired you to take up this practice in the first place. At the same time, while specific points of inner pain may be drawing you to mindfulness practice, it's important to understand how this works. Though you are inspired because you can see how practice will be of personal benefit, the *transformational experiences that come with mindfulness practice are a result of engaging in the simple protocol of mindfulness practice*, rather than something you seek directly. Mindfulness practice is a kindhearted, gentle practice that asks us to be attentive, without pushing too hard. It is the practice of returning the attention to simply paying attention—with patience, kindness, equanimity, and willingness—that creates the skills, openness of heart, and state of mind that invite transformative change. Connecting briefly with your "why" can help when you may be in the mood to do something else entirely than sit in practice.

Tomorrow, formal practice will include the next important element of setup: anchor.

🪷 Mindful Moment: Something You Already Know

Mindfulness is something we've all had a taste of at various moments in our lives. Have you ever spent time in nature—on a walk, or a run, or ambling with a friend—when suddenly, in the midst of it all, a feeling of complete relaxation, ease, or connection washes over you? This is the experience of mindful presence. Have you ever felt *right there*, present with your body, while in the middle of any athletic activity, when you are really connected with your physical experience and in "the zone"? Moment of mindfulness. How about while engaged in some artistic endeavor, painting, drawing, taking pictures—each detail of movement noted, purposeful? What about playing music, fully engaged in a writing flow, or creativity in any dimension? Or a sense of profound presence while simply playing fetch with your dog? Mindful moments. These are all authentic experiences of being mindful, and all of us have had some of them. Mindfulness makes us present—here, now. It's not something mysterious outside of us that we have to find. It is a capacity, a quality of presence, we already have for being mindful in the moment.

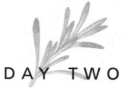

beginning practice: anchor

When you first become aware of something, there is a fleeting moment of pure awareness...just before you identify it...before you start thinking about it—before your mind says, "Oh, it's a dog." That flowing, soft-focused moment of pure awareness is mindfulness.

—HENEPOLA GUNARATANA

 MEDITATION PRACTICE: *2 minutes*

◁)) DAY TWO, *Anchor*

Today we'll add the next important element to your practice: anchor.

Setting Up Your Mindfulness Practice

Position

Begin by reestablishing position. Whether seated on a cushion on the floor or in a chair, let your position be upright and attentive, while at the same time comfortable, relaxed, and at ease.

Take a deep breath or two to help gather your attention and become aware of your body in the present moment. Feel your body on the cushion or chair.

Anchor

Once you are settled into position, find your anchor. With anchor, you begin to explore an important element of mindfulness practice: focused awareness. The natural movements of the breath are the anchor for beginning. The reason we focus on the feeling of the breath is because, for one, it takes place in the present moment. You can't breathe for yesterday, or tomorrow, for that matter. Breathing also takes place, for most of us, without any effort on our part. Breathing is also a neutral experience. We don't have a liking or disliking for it—it just happens. In essence, we are actually being breathed.

First, simply notice that your body is breathing. Feel the expansion and contraction of the belly, the rising and the falling of the chest as you breathe. Now, bring your attention to the breath where it enters and exits your nose. Can you feel the breath as it flows into and out of your nostrils? Any coolness, warmth, tingling, flow of other sensations, right beneath the nose? Because this area is more precise than anywhere else in your body for feeling the breath, it will be your anchor point, the object of your focused awareness, the point to which you return your attention as you start your mindfulness meditation practice.

Allow the breath to continue naturally, without trying to control it in any way. See if you can feel one breath at a time. Your only task is to stay attentive to the sensations of each in-and-out breath at the small area at and right beneath your nostrils. When your mind wanders, which it will, let go of that thought or feeling and return your focus to the breath, without reproach. In this way, meditation trains you to stay in the moment before you rather than rehashing the past or worrying about the future. It teaches you how to be gentle with yourself and with others, to pardon any lapses, and to move on.

During your practice, you may discover that your breathing rhythm changes—or not. Just allow it to be whatever it is, naturally.

🪷 Mindful Moment: Muddy Water

The best way to let muddy water clarify is to let it be still. This allows the sludge to settle. It is the same with your mind. Meditation gives you the opportunity and method for letting the mud in your mind sift out. With the energy of your attention—yet absent of force, or trying to push thoughts away—you invite the stillness by returning to anchor.

You may not even be aware of how much your mind is clouded with silt until you sit for mindfulness practice. You sit down and turn your attention inward, and the sound of a million disparate voices and static fills your head.

Whether you are aware of it or not, everything that happens to you makes an impression in your mind and body in some form—mentally as thought, emotion, or physical sensations in the body. Usually all of them. During the course of our busy days, we get so caught up in the details of living that often the issues with which we are dealing are not thoroughly processed. They become lodged in the unconscious and take on a life of their own. Then we wonder where all the tension and anxiety came from. The same tension and anxiety that drives us to fly off the handle, pound down the chips, or zone out online.

Mindfulness practice is your golden opportunity to allow all of this to process—without reactivity, repression, pushing it away, pretending it isn't there, or stirring up the mud in some other fashion. Your willingness to be present with what is? This is what allows the silt to settle and clarity to be restored.

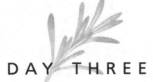

beginning practice: intention and remindfulness

A thought is not a fact—a thought is just a thought.
—JON KABAT-ZINN

MEDITATION PRACTICE: *3 minutes*

DAY THREE, *Intention and Remindfulness*

Today, we will add the next two steps of setting up formal mindfulness practice with PAIR: intention and remindfulness.

Intention and Remindfulness

Position

Whichever position you have chosen, let it be dignified and attentive, while comfortable at the same time. Breathe deeply once or twice to help gather your attention. Become aware of your body and how the body feels, sitting on the chair or floor.

Anchor

Find your anchor point at the base of the nostrils, the area that gives the most focused connection with the sensation of the breath. Remember, in mindfulness of breath practice, your task is to simply be with the natural in-and-out flow of the breath. There is no need to alter the breath in any way. The key to mindfulness of breath is to actually *feel* the breath at anchor point while staying at ease, rather than visualizing the breath, thinking about where it is going, or making your breathing a cerebral process. Just be aware of the physical sensations of the breath coming and going. This brings you mindfully right into the present.

Intention

Set the intention of sitting in continuous practice today for three minutes. If you become slightly uncomfortable, take note and see if you can remain still, bringing your attention back to the breath. If you become deeply uncomfortable, however, such as experiencing pain in your legs or knees, it is okay to gently, mindfully adjust your position and start again.

Just as important is the intention of attitude that you bring to your sitting practice. Kindness, patience, nonjudgment, a sense of relaxation, and a willingness to be present with whatever arises are the qualities to cultivate.

Remindfulness

It's likely that your mind has already started to wander. In fact, all sorts of things will come into your mind when you sit for practice. If that's the case, you're not doing anything wrong. It's actually quite normal. Many distractions will arise—a steady parade of thoughts, mental images, bodily itches, plans, or emotions. You may not even notice this wandering until you have been lost in thought for a while, engaged in planning or excavating a remembrance.

The instant you become aware that your attention has wandered, even if you don't notice it until you've been running with a story in your mind for some time, gently return your attention to anchor. Adopt an attitude of compassion and friendliness toward your mind. After all, it is only doing what it has been allowed to do for the last several years—decades even. It's a good thinker!

You may feel that it's impossible for you to keep the mind still or that you'll never get the hang of getting the mind quiet—and how on earth can you train the mind in the midst of all this commotion? It is helpful to understand that the important thing here is not that you shouldn't have any thoughts. You are practicing letting go of thoughts and returning to the point of concentration, every time you realize you've wandered off to thinking. This is what mindfulness training is all about—the return of the attention, not the absence of thought.

It doesn't matter how often wandering mind happens. As soon as you notice that your mind has wandered, you have already **remembered** your intention. Gently let go of thoughts, and kindly **return** your attention to the present via the actual physical feeling of the breath, your anchor. **Repeat** this every time you discover that your attention has wandered. *Remember, return, repeat.* Collectively, we'll call this *remindfulness.* This simple act—beginning over and over again—is the essential art of mindfulness meditation practice. You simply begin again. Gently. Patiently. As a matter of fact, it's not about the breath as much as the attention and attitude. Feeling the breath is simply your tool for gathering your awareness and attention while practicing equanimity.

When the time is up, gently open your eyes. Set an intention to bring some of this quality of mindfulness to the present moment forward with you into your day.

Think Much?

How did today's practice go? Did you notice your mind wanted to plan, remember, muse, worry, fantasize, tell itself stories—basically wander all over the place and do anything but be present with the breath? To reassure you, this is what everyone experiences as they get started with mindfulness practice. These activities are the habits of the mind. After all, we have spent our entire lives developing mental habits that are completely contradictory to uninterrupted mindfulness. Thinking is what our minds do—try simply "not thinking" for a few seconds, and you'll see what I mean. This is why we have the anchor, the breath, to use during meditation practice. It gives the mind a point around which to rally its overenthusiastic resources.

Some sources tell us we have tens of thousands of thoughts a day. Thoughts come unbidden—arising out of our control. There's nothing inherently wrong with thoughts. The human ability to plan ahead, learn from the past, troubleshoot, and strategize is one of our best features. It has been a critical player in our survival.

But we all know the downside of this marvelous capability of our minds. While thinking can be the source of much of our brilliance, it is also the root of much of our pain. Thoughts can become exhaustingly circuitous. They can darken our experience with needless negativity and fear. With them we borrow trouble from the future and replay past regrets—ad nauseam.

Thoughts quickly take on a life of their own by becoming stories— stories that our minds run with. Excessive rumination, tumbling a drama over and over again in our minds, saps our strength, wastes our precious time, destroys the moment, builds a mountain of anxiety, and temporarily drives us nuts. For example, this morning I woke up with a slight headache. I rarely have headaches, so when a headache would show up, I'll see if I can find a possible cause. I thought back to what I'd had to eat the day before that might have been the culprit, but I could find nothing out of the ordinary. I decided to see if my headache didn't just dissipate on its own and settled into my morning meditation. Before I knew it, my mind was off and running. I thought of how my aunt had experienced a brain hemorrhage decades ago, and how the first sign for her had been a headache. I started imagining best internet key words to search—"headache + brain hemorrhage." From there, I jumped to possible hospital scenarios. What did my current health plan cover, and would I be able to be easily admitted in an emergency, and darn that new health plan anyway, it's so complex and pricey, and how far down the road until I qualify for Medicare, and can I apply for it online when the time comes? Rumination bordering on catastrophizing.

Certainly, analyzing my health plan is a smart thing to do, but was predawn the best time for such investigations? I would have been bet- ter off leaving the "story" right after a review of my eats the day before and getting back to the rest at a better time. As it turned out, I soon noticed that my mind had wandered away from this internal minidrama to something else. I brought my attention back to my anchor—remindfulness—the headache soon dissolved, and that was that.

These habits of our mind—that part that runs with story, imagines the worst, and endlessly fantasizes about possible outcomes—pulls us from our present experience with serious side effects. Where do you think those unsettling emotions we were just talking about—anxiety, anger, guilt, fear, sadness, nervousness—often get their start?

It doesn't matter how many thoughts pop into your mind each day—it's what you do with them that matters. Mindfulness meditation introduces a revolutionary concept regarding your brain and your thoughts: namely, that you have thoughts, *but your thoughts are not who you are*. We are so used to identifying with them—following the story of each one that arises and believing everything they say—is it any wonder that our minds and emotions are all over the place?

Mindfulness Opens a New Space

The practice of mindfulness meditation allows you to create a space between awareness and the thoughts that arise. In the process of opening this space, you learn to discriminate your sense of self and identity from your thoughts. You become able to see your thoughts as mental processes rather than a fully accurate snapshot of reality. You slowly shift from thinking and becoming immersed in the mind's stories over and over again to another mode that will serve you better: awareness itself.[1] This ultimately supports you in becoming less reactive and more intentional in your actions. You experience greater equanimity, giving rise to a fresh ability to be more discriminating in your choices and responses. This ability to choose is the cornerstone of change. The mental muscle you strengthen by continuing to bring your awareness back to your anchor point in formal practice is the same one that allows you to keep your hand out of the cookie jar or from blurting out regretfully in an argument with your spouse.

✿ Mindful Moment: Mental Noting

When your mind repeatedly wanders during practice, it can be helpful to implement what is known as mental noting. Mental noting is a strategy that uses a small degree of thinking to help you let thoughts go by during mindfulness practice. This keeps your mind happy by giving it something to do in the interests of the greater picture—letting go of compelling thoughts rather than getting caught up in them. Thoughts actually arise in the present—yet most of our thoughts are about the past or the future, taking us away from the present moment. With mental noting, you are utilizing in-the-present thinking to keep you centered. It is also a simple, effective way to develop concentration.

The instructions for mental noting are simple. As you begin your practice, the first thought that comes down the tracks you can meet with a mental note of "thinking." This simple step creates space for you to let go of the thought. By noting "thinking," you acknowledge the thought without judgment, pushing it away, or diminishing its importance. After all, thoughts of making an important phone call, paying bills, doing your daily exercise, or restocking the fridge are certainly important. But you can deal with them later—sometimes, in just another ten or fifteen minutes. *Right now* is not the time—since this is the time you have set aside for mindfulness practice.

Mental noting is done as a silent whisper in your mind—very softly, gently, in the background. Without force. When noting, do it as soon as you notice a thought arising so that the noting (aware) mind is continuously present as much as possible. For the next thought, do the same. And the next, and the next. You may find that you have been lost in thought for five or ten minutes before you are aware of it. And you may be surprised at how quickly this simple process allows thoughts to pass on by, without you diving into them.

If you are having an unusually tough job of staying with your anchor of the breath, mental noting can serve as ballast to the present and to reestablish mindfulness. This gives the mind something to do in a way that supports meditation rather than distracts from it. Maintaining kindness and a quiet inner voice—no yelling—is important. Keep it friendly and use a light touch, only calling upon it as needed or as you see helpful.

I use mental noting when I am feeling particularly distracted. It can be very effective at helping bring greater focus to my meditation in these circumstances. Usually, I let go of the strategy after it has done its job. I'll pick it up again if necessary. There are no rules about it, or a requirement to use it. See if mental noting helps you, and if not, then that's fine, too.

Staying with your experience—the breath as anchor during formal practice, implementing simple tools such as mental noting to keep you connected with your experience, and returning your attention to the point of anchor—actively shapes your mind. Growing your awareness of the mind's tendencies and habits strengthens your ability to choose how to respond in the moment outside of formal practice. Meditation is about befriending your thinking, holding it gently in awareness, and letting go of thoughts—rather than shutting them off or changing them.

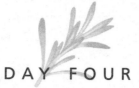

DAY FOUR

am i doing it "right"?

*It's very nice and helpful to become calm and peaceful, but in
mindfulness meditation, we don't hold that up as the great goal.
The goal is to pay attention.*

—GIL FRONSDAL, Insight Meditation Teacher

MEDITATION PRACTICE: *4 minutes*

DAY FOUR, *Meditation on Breath*

You may, like many of us, embark on a meditation practice with
an expectation of the kind of inner experience you should be having. This
can be accompanied by a judgment about whether or not you are "doing it
right."

Am I Doing It Right?

Your experiences during practice are not a measure of whether or not you
are practicing correctly. During some meditations you may experience
great spaciousness, happiness, and a sense of peace. Other times you will
feel agitated, impatient, and desirous of doing anything but sitting there.

Sometimes your mind is just more active than at other times, your emotions more turbulent. These can show up during practice time. Often there will be no apparent reason that you find it easier to focus one day more than another. And sometimes you'll have what feels like a terrible sitting practice—then abide in a calm, openhearted spaciousness the rest of the day. It doesn't matter. The important thing is to practice anyway. This underscores the importance of devoting attention to your practice. The valuable moments spent in practice help you to process the ebbs and flows of life, giving you tools for living with more equanimity.

Mindfulness practice is actually very simple. In our enthusiasm for getting it right, we can overthink the task. And overthinking things is one of our problems.

The Golden Moment

Desiring one type of experience and rejecting another during practice misses the point. It is important to cultivate an accepting friendliness toward the whole meditative process. Rather than harboring some kind of ideal about your mind being perfectly still and unwavering, try a more realistic, kinder approach. Every moment of remembering and returning, coupled with awareness and equanimity, is very important and transforming. It is actually the designated task, for the foundation of mindfulness meditation is repeatedly returning the attention to your anchor while training your mind to reside in balance—an equanimity that transfers directly to time outside of formal practice. One of my teachers calls this point of remindfulness the "golden moment." It doesn't matter how many times you find yourself lost in thought. Simply bring your attention gently back to anchor as soon as you know it has wandered. Remindfulness is the currency of practice. When you look at it this way, the more your mind wanders, the more practice you are getting!

Absolute stillness may happen from time to time, but knowing that it is the nature of the mind to wander makes a big difference in how you approach practice. As you become more experienced, it will generally become easier to let go of thoughts and distractions. Rather than trying to produce a particular state or to change what you are feeling in any way, simply notice each thought, feeling, and sensation that comes up.

Your willingness to be with whatever is presenting itself—and repeatedly returning to anchor, with kindness and patience—is all that you need for practice.

Tips for Helping You Focus during Formal Practice

In addition to mental noting, here are some other simple strategies that may help you get focused during practice. If you need a little assist staying disentangled from thoughts, you might try these.

One Breath at a Time

See if it is possible to sustain your attention at anchor point over the course of one entire inhalation or one entire exhalation. Then see if you can sustain the attention over the entire course of one full breath, including the natural pause between inhalation and exhalation.

The Train Station

During mindfulness meditation practice, remember that your task is not to block or suppress thoughts—or to try not to have any thoughts at all. Accept that thoughts are going to come on their own. It's part of the human condition. The difference is that with mindfulness practice you are becoming trained and skilled in thought management: how you engage with them, where you go with them, and finding out about their power to drag your anchor all over the place as you get, quite literally, lost in thought.

A very helpful device for getting some perspective on the activity of the mind is the train station analogy. It can help you gain skill in managing your runaway thinking mind so that you can be more present and revolutionize reactivity. Imagine that you are standing in a train station. Your capacity of mind to be aware—of anything, including thoughts—is the station platform. Your stream of thoughts—mental images, memories, ideas about the future—is the train coming down the tracks. As it rolls into the station, you have a choice. You can either jump onto the train—get caught up in a thought—or stay at the platform.

Our habit is to get onto the train. Sometimes we find ourselves ten miles down the tracks before we even realize we jumped on board. If, instead, you remain mindful—aware of the thought train coming down the tracks and your capacity to let it chug on by—you can stay at the platform. The thought shows up, but instead of getting caught up in it, you understand that you have the freedom to *not* board that train.

Translated directly to your mindfulness practice? There is a difference between being aware of a thought and *thinking* a thought. With practice, you will become increasingly aware of thoughts arriving and departing—without you getting caught up in all of them. As you become more experienced, you will detect these "trains" at earlier and earlier points in time. Eventually, you will even be able to sense them coming from a distance way down the tracks as an approaching energy, enabling you to let them pass easily, almost effortlessly. By the way, this skill of being able to choose thoughts or let them go by translates directly to the eating experience.

Sounds: Distraction or Reminder?

Sounds that come to your ears during your formal practice time can be experienced as a distraction or annoyance. I've developed another way to look at it that shifts the auditory experience. When a sound intrudes upon the quiet—the cooing of a dove, the water heater starting up, the sounds of activity in another part of the house—I use it as an opportunity for remindfulness, to pull the wandering mind back to anchor. This simple shift in attitude about sounds during practice has been very helpful, sometimes returning me to anchor more often than I might experience otherwise. After all, sounds we hear are current events! This means they have the quality of bringing us right back to the present moment.

☙ Mindful Moment: Sharon's Mindfulness Journey

Sharon is a health coach who also teaches healthy vegan cooking classes. A busy mother with three teens, she finds meditation practice to be of significant support to sustainability of her work and busy life:

I began meditating regularly a few years ago after a week-end retreat with an oncologist who left medicine because he found he could help more patients with meditation than with medication. In his course, I learned the physiological way that meditation works to release stress in the brain created by our memories.

As a result of practicing, I'm much more grounded and less affected by stress on a physical and emotional level. This helps me keep moving along the path that leads me to my desired goal of being able to spread the word about how eating a vegan/whole food plant-based diet can prevent and reverse disease. I, like many others, have a very active mind that tends to jump around and can be quite resistant to quieting. But my daily meditation practice has strengthened my ability to let go, much as lifting weights has strengthened my muscles. I have learned not to try to quiet the thoughts when they inevitably come, but to simply observe them, without reacting to them, and to gently guide my mind back. With meditation in place, I am much more peaceful internally, and I always know I have a safe haven to turn to when making challenging decisions or taking steps that are outside of my comfort zone. I recommend meditation to all of my health coaching clients who are working on lifestyle improvements, because I know it helps them manage stress and make choices on a daily basis that are completely in line with their goals.

Meditation keeps me from getting ruffled when encountering people who tell me they could never eat like me, yet they are clearly struggling with their health. I find myself feeling much more compassionate towards them and encouraging them to just take one step and see if they notice a difference. Even if I get push-back, I'm able to stay calm and share my truth in a non-judgmental way, which would undoubtedly be much more of a challenge if I was not in tune with that inner voice.[1]

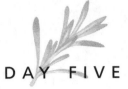

DAY FIVE

wandering mind, unhappy mind?

I've had a lot of worries in my life, most of which never happened.

—MARK TWAIN

 MEDITATION PRACTICE: *5 minutes*

🔊 DAY FIVE, *Training a Puppy*

💡 For those who undertake a practice of mindfulness, it doesn't take long before you realize just how wildly unruly the mind can be. What sounds so simple—gather your attention and put it where you want—presents such a challenge! What are the mechanisms in place that keep thoughts running as they do?

Default Mode Network

If you could take a peek under the hood and see what is going on in your brain, you would discover, along with the brain's other brilliant assets and capabilities, what brain researchers call our default mode network (DMN). The default mode is so named because it is where mental activity settles when your mind is not focused on a task. The DMN is characterized by—surprise, surprise—mind-wandering. It is in this default mode that we recollect memories, envision the future, fantasize, daydream, ruminate, and experience thoughts and feelings that are unrelated to events in the here and now.[1] The DMN is also known as the narrative network—for when you just let the mind wander as is its habit, it is largely caught up in stories about yourself. As you undertake mindfulness practice, you begin to become aware of this aspect of the mind that you may not have been wise to before.

Apparently, along with the important capabilities the default mode network brings, this activity has a downside. How could something that sounds so innocent be at the same time problematic for your happiness?

Is a Wandering Mind an Unhappy Mind?

We typically spend about 50 percent of our time in the mind-wandering zone, according to the largest study on mind-wandering states and happiness research conducted to date.[2] This Harvard study contains nearly a quarter of a million samples from about five thousand people from eighty-three different countries. Data was collected to find out how mind-wandering relates to happiness. Study subjects were pulled from a widely varied population, ranging in age from eighteen to eighty-eight and collectively representing eighty-six major occupational categories.

According to the study, people were no happier, and often substantially less happy, when their minds were wandering than when they were not—*no matter what they were doing at the time or to where their minds wandered*. This held true whether they were doing something they enjoyed or doing something they didn't enjoy. It held true even if their mind wandered to thoughts of an activity more enjoyable than that with which they were engaged. Consistently, mind-wandering diminished happiness.

For example, commuting to work is not an activity people reported as liking very much. Yet people were substantially happier when they were focused on their commute as opposed to letting their mind wander off to something else during that time. You might not enjoy doing the dishes, and assume that fantasizing about being on the beach in Hawaii might increase your happiness. According to the research, you are happier being mindfully present doing the dishes than slogging through the suds with your thoughts on Waikiki. This pattern held true for every activity the study measured. So though negative moods are known to cause mind-wandering, the study results strongly suggested that mind-wandering is generally the cause, and not merely the consequence, of unhappiness.

And is it any surprise, really, once you think about it? Reliving the past—and other default-mode-network cohorts—brings to mind the most common culprits of mental unrest: anxiety (over potential presents or imagined futures), depression (over regretted pasts or troubling presents), or obsessive thinking about . . . well, just about anything. Mind-wandering hooks up with other neural activity in the default mode network that can pull us into endless rumination. It's here in the default zone that we can also get caught up in a craving, or in obsessively defending a viewpoint—like a dog defending a bone.

More than one study has linked activity in brain regions that are major cofactors in the default mode network—the playground of daydreaming and mind-wandering—and the role they play in addiction.[3] Default-mode-network activity has been associated with processes ranging from anxiety to lapses in attention, major depression, clinical disorders such as attention deficit hyperactivity disorder (ADHD), and even Alzheimer's disease.[4] Perhaps it should come as no surprise that too much time in the default mode is associated with lower levels of happiness.

It's not that the DMN doesn't serve a good purpose. We need it to plan projects, to reflect upon the past to improve our future, to synthesize information, and for other essentials for living. Yet though the default network is a remarkable evolutionary achievement that allows you to evaluate, reason, and plan, spending too much time there can have an emotional cost and drain your energy. Think about all those times when you have been plagued by replaying a regret over and over in your mind, wishing you could shake it because it is coloring your entire outlook. All those times you've spent obsessing over a future event, catastrophizing, imagining the worst. All the time you may have spent mentally rehashing your food or fitness plan. If you've ever surfed the internet (which is not unlike the default mode network, with its ability to pull us into one related topic after another until we forgot what we were looking for in the first place) and been left with a feeling of mild burnout coupled with sadness, you've simply hitched up the nomadic nature of the DMN with tech support.

If the research tells us that too much time hanging out in the default zone can be problematic, what does it tell us about an alternative? While we benefit from some aspects of wandering mind, how might we offset or circumvent the downsides of processes that are subcomponents of the default mode network—such as getting caught up in obsessive thought patterns and cravings?

Wouldn't it be nice if you could move more freely between the default network and a place of greater well-being, happiness, and peace?

Tomorrow: mindfulness as antidote to getting mired in the dark side of the default mode network.

🪷 Mindful Moment: Training a Puppy

One of my meditation teachers, Jack Kornfield, has said that working with the breath is a bit like training a puppy. You pick the puppy up, set them down on the paper, and tell them to stay. But does the puppy stay? Nope. Just like the mind, the puppy gets up, wanders around, and follows a million scents in a million directions. Not unlike your attention and thoughts. So you pick the puppy (attention) up again, put the puppy down on the paper (the breath) once again, and tell them to stay. Given enough time and loving attention, the puppy begins to figure things out. We may be a tad slower than puppies in this regard, but it is still possible to train the mind, as impossible as it may seem at the start.

Using the example of training a puppy, we all know that it is not a good idea to scold or beat the puppy when it strays. Keep in mind that an important element of mindfulness is the willingness to be present, without judgment. Translated to your mindfulness practice, when you find yourself thinking judgmental thoughts such as "I'll never get this right" or "I just can't do this mindfulness thing!" to respond by berating yourself doesn't help. It only adds another diversion and makes you feel bad by spiraling you into the DMN. Instead of practicing mindfulness, you're practicing judgment and blame. And what you practice grows stronger.

Just pick the puppy up by bringing the attention back to the breath. Try to stay present, attentively, for the next breath or two. When the mind wanders off, bring it back again, with kindness and patience. Gradually, with practice, returning to anchor will become easier. You will more often be able to stay present with the breath for longer periods of time. Translated to living, this means you will be able to abide less in the wandering mind and more in the present. This gives you more and more opportunities to see that you need not default to old habits that drive your thoughts and emotions on autopilot. You gain the freedom that awareness brings. You can reclaim the only moment you really have—this one.

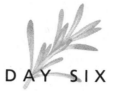

must be present to win

*Each of us possesses the potential needed to free ourselves from
the mental states that perpetuate our own suffering and that
of others—the potential to find inner peace for ourselves and
contribute to the happiness of all beings.*

—MATTHIEU RICARD

MEDITATION PRACTICE: *6 minutes*

DAY SIX, *Meditation on the Breath*

Finding out about the default mode network of the brain
can't help but reframe your ideas about what's going on in your mind.
Remember, the default mode isn't the number-one bad guy. After all, it
helps you plan tasks, reflect upon your past actions, and connect the
dots of your experiences. Yet some of its functions can also deliver a
big dose of downer. Being wary of its runaway forces—highly correlated with obsessive thinking, cravings, anxiety, and negative mood
states—makes good sense. It gives you a decided new interest in managing what's going on up there. Today we'll further explore brain states,
mindfulness meditation, and neuroplasticity.

Snap Out of It!

Focused awareness practice—as you are engaged in with meditation on the breath—can be seen as mental training to reduce the competitive distraction and daydreaming activities of the DMN. By bringing your awareness to the present-moment experience, mindfulness pulls you out of the mind-wandering state. It simultaneously switches off brain activity in the default mode network. It's actually impossible for them to run concurrently, like diverting a train to another track. Any time you are "on task," tightly focusing your brain on a specific activity— whether parallel parking or immersed in a good book—activity in the default zone idles down.

When we're craving, when we're anxious, when we're thinking obsessively, when we're getting in our own way in one way or another, as occurs with increased default-network[1] recruitment, that part of the brain associated with these states—the posterior cingulated cortex (PCC)—gets activated. When we look at functional magnetic resonance imaging (fMRI) taken when someone is sitting in meditation practice and observe what is taking place from moment to moment, there is a distinct difference in the imaging depending on how attentive to meditation the person is. When ruminative mental states (mind-wandering) are being experienced, there is increased activity in the PCC. When focused in meditation practice, activity is decreased in the PCC and stepped up in regions of the brain associated with cognitive control.[2] This difference is even detected in something as subtle as *thinking about* the breath (ruminative) versus actually *feeling* the breath physically (present-moment experience).[3] In our penchant for reward-based learning, wouldn't it be great if we could hook up to fMRI when we sit for practice and actually see the difference we are making in our well-being because of the impact mindfulness meditation has on our brains?

Mindfulness meditation teaches you how to switch from wandering to attentive awareness of your present-moment experience directly— anywhere, any time. In a fraction of a second, as you mindfully direct your attention to being fully present in real time, you disengage from default thoughts, habits, and undesirable behavior patterns of the ruminative network such as cravings and anxiety.

How might this play out in your experience? Let's take craving as an example. Typically, you might either get caught up in a craving or find yourself struggling against it in usual fashion: brooding about why you should or shouldn't indulge in the substance or behavior, fearing what might happen if you do, or replaying the horrors of last time you did. While learning from past cavings to cravings is helpful information, you are instead probably caught up in your usual spiral of should and shouldn't. This not only fails to deliver a resolution, it also creates enormous inner struggle and personal angst. It's not as if it's a new song—it's an old tune that has most likely played a gazillion times in your mind.

With mindfulness, you disarm the inner war. You turn your attention from your default battle zone to the breath and notice what your body feels like. Neurologically, you've just turned the switch off in the default mode network. Yet rather than running away from the situation, you walk through the middle of it. You've done it in a way that keeps you connected with your current experience. This is in contrast to denying it or suppressing it, which only comes back to haunt you later. Here, you are neither joining with the cravings nor fighting them.

With acceptance and curiosity, and a willingness to be present, you observe the qualities of craving itself. What is the experience actually like, physically and mentally, to crave? It may be felt as agitation, restlessness, tension, or a longing that accompanies the thought of the thing, substance, food, or experience that is the object of your craving. For example, if you are craving strawberry ice cream, the ice cream is the *target* of craving, and how your body and mind feel are the *feelings* of the craving experience. By teasing apart the experience of craving in this fashion, you begin to realize that these are actually two phenomena. Instead of getting hijacked by the craving, or trying to distract yourself from it—thus reinforcing the craving loop—it is here that you have the opportunity to initiate a different response. More on cravings on Day Twenty-Five (page 200).

The Benefits of Being Present

Through this process of engaging mindful attention, you open up the space for self-regulation of thoughts, emotions, and behaviors—qualities long associated with well-being and the cornerstone of change.[4] You begin to see thoughts and feelings, such as cravings, as objects. You gain insights into your behavior patterns. You give yourself a ticket to that space between stimulus and response—that interval in which you can make a different choice, enhancing everything from personal well-being and health to your interpersonal relationships and conversations with everyone from your kid to your coworker. You bring more clarity and vividness to present-moment experiences, contributing to your freedom and happiness in a direct way.

Neuroplasticity and Mindfulness: What You Practice Grows Stronger

Your mind is what your brain does. And what you do with your mind, in turn, shapes your brain. When you learn something new, due to neuroplasticity, your brain changes structure to adapt to the demands.[5] For example, taxi drivers—expert navigators in their own right—have larger posterior hippocampi, a brain structure important for spatial representation of the environment. It's not that people with bigger posterior hippocampi sign up to be cabbies—it comes as a result of their extensive navigational experience driving taxi cabs. It is a task-oriented adaptation via neuroplasticity.[6]

When it comes to mindfulness, the growth and change we see in the brain is specific to the processes of mindfulness practice that has been called positive neuroplasticity. In mindfulness meditation, you practice self-regulation of attention, in which you engage focused attention on an object, such as the feeling of the breath. You continue to monitor and regulate the quality of your attention, bringing awareness and attention together over and over again. By cultivating a specific orientation to your experience, you cultivate self-regulation of reactivity.[7]

With continued practice these benefits of mindfulness become part of your inner landscape. In brain research, mindfulness meditators show increased thickness in areas of the brain associated with emotional and mental processing, proof positive that when it comes to mental activity, what you practice grows stronger.[8] These changes translate into increased ability to more successfully navigate stressful situations throughout your day.

And the default mode network? Advanced practitioners have an especially acute ability to notice when the mind has wandered. Over time, researchers believe that meditation practice transforms the resting-state experience into one that resembles a meditative state—a more present-centered mode characterized by decreased anxiety, stress, cravings, depression, and other disquieting states. You create a new normal of awareness, reduced reactivity, and self-regulation of response. In other words, meditators have a new default mode. This plays out in reduced mind-wandering—not only during, but outside formal meditation practice time.[9]

☙ Mindful Moment: Moving More Mindfulness into Your Day

Making a connection between your formal mindfulness and living more mindfully during the rest of your day takes practice. We are quite used to being lost on autopilot and in the default zone whenever not attending to specific tasks. Being more mindful with day-to-day tasks will take a little practice before it becomes more naturally integrated into your day.

As a tool to increase moments of mindfulness, it can help to have prompts that remind you. This can be especially true as you are getting started with mindfulness practice, as it helps you bring a new thread of mindfulness into your day.

1. Set an awareness timer. Each time the timer sounds, you note gently in what zone you are playing. Are you on a task at work, mindfully engaged? Are you doing the dishes, dreaming of Waikiki? Are you lost in thought? Are you on a walk, engaged in the beauties of nature or good conversation? Are you in the midst of a good run, completely enthralled in "the zone"? Remember, mindfulness means awareness—and becoming aware of our habits of mind throughout the day is an excellent feedback tool.

   While writing this book, I downloaded a program to my computer that sounds a chime every fifteen minutes to bring me back to mindfulness. Every time this charming bell sound rings, it prompts me to refresh mindful awareness. The overall effect is a more focused, productive, and relaxed writing experience.

2. Connect mindfulness with a task. It could be brushing your teeth, getting in the car to go to work, taking the dog for a walk, doing the dishes, making the morning coffee or tea, getting out of bed after waking up, or lying down to go to sleep at night. Pick an activity that you do every day at a specific time, and establish it as a designated daily opportunity to simply check in with your state of mind. During the activity, bring your focus on the sensations of what you are doing: body movements, taste, touch, smells, sights, and sounds. Do you feel relaxed and at ease, or is your body poised for fight, freeze, or flight? Are your shoulders tight? Do you feel tension in your face, your stomach? Simply observe. No need to do anything with it, push it away, or give it any deep meaning. You are simply practicing getting better at the mind-body connection. This growing connection and awareness with physical sensations allows you to inhabit your body and mind in a new way.

After a few days, you can add another daily activity, then another. Notice as thoughts arise during this activity. Just as in formal practice, acknowledge them, and bring your attention back to the meal, the walking of the dog, the brushing of your teeth. Should boredom or frustration arise, acknowledge it, and bring your attention back to the task. Again and again, your attention will wander—that is the nature of the mind. With kindness and patience, simply employ "R"—remindfulness.

Gradually, with intention and practice, staying mindfully present more often during your day will be possible. Being mindful simply means that mind and body are in the same place, rather than letting the mind run off into its usual wandering while the body does something else. When you wash dishes, wash dishes. When you eat, eat. This makes "when you meditate, meditate" easier. These practices help us to let go of thoughts that drag us into negative mental states, making our lives less stressful and filling them with greater comfort. *What you practice grows stronger.*

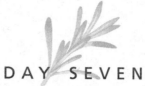

bodily sensations

Your body is not there just to carry around your head. The research findings indicate that we need to start thinking about how the mind manifests itself in various parts of the body and, beyond that, how we can bring that process into consciousness.

—CANDACE PERT, PhD, *Molecules of Emotion: The Science Behind Mind-Body Medicine*

MEDITATION PRACTICE: *7 minutes*

DAY SEVEN, *Meditation on the Breath*

Devoting these minutes every day exclusively to mindfulness practice is the foundation of mindful living. By practicing every day, you develop concentration coupled with awareness. It doesn't mean that your mind is quiet or that thoughts no longer intrude. A silent mind is not what you are seeking to achieve. Rather, you are developing the ability to observe your habits of thinking and sharpening the tools of attentive awareness. You are discovering that you do not need to hop on each thought that comes down the tracks—that you do have some say in the matter. You are expanding that space between stimulus and response on purpose. This gives you the tools for living more mindfully and allows you to enjoy the benefits that come with it.

Today, you'll discover the important connection between mindfulness and bodily sensations. This will give purpose and meaning to the addition of meditation on bodily sensations to your practice tomorrow.

The Mind-Body Connection

Whether you are aware of it or not, every thought you have has a corresponding sensation in your body. These sensations, just like the breath, are taking place in the present moment. Often, a thought will even arise first as a physical sensation. Sometimes it is the other way around. And sometimes physical sensations arise without a thought component to them, such as when you stub your toe or slip into a warm bath.

Why Is Mindfulness of Bodily Sensations Helpful?

It's no accident that the word *feeling* is used for mental and emotional, as well as tactile, experiences. Even when we are not consciously aware of our feelings, we still react to them. This reactivity can leave a trail of tension that plays itself out in a multitude of ways—as mindless eating, the bowl of ice cream "because I deserve it," the gobbled bag of chips, the surprising outburst of anger, troubling anxiety, inexplicable sadness, a compulsion to check your email.

As you bring attention to the physical sensations in your body with mindfulness practice, you experience your feelings directly. Mindfulness practice steps up both your *interoceptive* and *somatosensory* awareness. Interoception includes your internal visceral sensations and sensations of breathing—often laden with emotion. Numerous studies have identified interoception as a central mechanism of mindfulness training for facilitating emotional and cognitive self-regulation. Interoception is also key to eating mindfully, in harmony with your hunger and fullness signals.

Somatosensation is conscious perception of touch, temperature, pressure, pain, and vibration. Sharpening both interoception and somatosensation brings previously unnoticed sensations in your body into conscious awareness.[1] This is profoundly useful because it reveals the intimate connections between what you are feeling in the body, emotions, and runaway trains of thought. You find out a lot more about how you are reacting to thoughts, emotions, and what is going on around you. By placing your attention on these sensations, you are able to access more directly what is driving your behaviors as it helps to free you from the mental story lines—the dramas, judgments, and projections—around them. Without the stories distracting you, you forge a fresh pathway for changing habits of reactivity. You are able to bring to light what might otherwise remain obscured, dismantling the negative forces of hidden obstacles. Mindfulness of these bodily sensations also makes it possible for you to better detect and regulate when the mind wanders from focus, leading to enhanced self-regulation of thought and emotion.

Mindfulness gives you the tools to navigate these physical sensations and the thoughts and emotions to which they are linked. When you are disconnected from your physical experience, you lose touch with your inner experience. Consciously reconnecting with bodily sensations helps you to discover buried thoughts and emotions. Think of them as the voice of your unconscious mind. Reactivity to these thoughts and emotions may be showing up in ways that cause you a great deal of pain, such as baffling eating behaviors and patterns of dealing with other people. It works the other way, too. Ignoring, suppressing, or wishing away aspects of your emotional and mental experience disconnects you from your body—the physical manifestation of your experiences. Reestablishing this connectivity with your body leads to a greater capacity to respond to the world with healthy emotions, greater clarity, good intentions, and positive motivations. You move from reactivity to living more consciously responsive, to living with greater ease and happiness.

Just as you are cultivating nonreactivity to the stream of thoughts that present themselves in the mindfulness of breath meditation, mindfulness of bodily sensations is another way to simply be present with your experience. Often our automatic preferences and judgments get in the way of our ability to know what is actually taking place as we run everything through a filter of previous experience. A deeper understanding of your habits of reactivity gives you the possibility of choosing a fresh response. Being nonreactively present for your physical experience goes a long way in learning to do so with the rest of your life. You experience growing freedom from getting entangled in the thought processes that carry you away with stories and imaginings.

One of my first experiences of bodily awareness creating new responsiveness was demonstrated to me in dramatic fashion the very day that my initial ten-day mindfulness retreat came to a close. My parents had picked me up at the airport to transport me from the retreat to meeting my husband for a planned trip. Mom, Dad, and I stopped at a diner for a bite to eat. Sitting down, waiting for the food to arrive, I became acutely aware of the world of reactions that inhabited my mind and body when it came to my parents. I possessed a troubling reactivity to my dad that I had been aware of for years. I was always poised to judge what he had to say and was aware of my tendency to counterpoint him, often for no apparent reason other than to play out some sort of rebellion. Who knows why. It doesn't really matter. But what did matter is that it had been affecting our relationship for a long time. And I didn't know how to do differently. I'd tried being more patient, not letting him "get under my skin." But I never could figure out how.

This time, internally, I opened into what I had been practicing for the ten days of retreat. I decided to simply be present with Dad. What if I were to be authentically interested in and listen to what he had to say—as if he were someone that I hadn't built a wall of reactivity toward? As I listened to him, I was acutely aware of my old patterns and responses. I turned my attention to where I could feel them in my body: tension in my belly, a tightening in my chest. I could hear them in my head—in an entirely new way, as the qualities of mental reactivity became so clear. Yet this time, staying mindfully present and aware of all of it, I was able to navigate right through these as simply old worn-out shoes that I didn't need anymore and to be genuinely present with and attentive to Dad. I had one of the best times of my life with him because of this one simple shift. It was astonishing and freeing, and a very happy experience. Over the years, I still had on and off struggles with talking with Dad. But from that moment at the diner nothing was quite the same. It had ushered in a new way of being with my father that I never imagined possible.

Learning to move out of automaticity is the core of mindfulness. This is not the same as trying to analyze why you feel as you do, where in the heck you got this or that pattern of reactivity, or why you are the poster child for the problems of being the middle child. It's quite easy to get caught up in trying to figure out why we are thinking or feeling a certain way. Though these analyses can be helpful processes on their own—as an adjunct to mindfulness—meandering in this manner is not your aim during mindfulness practice. Thinking itself can become a barrier to understanding.

Tomorrow, we'll add mindfulness meditation of bodily sensations to your formal mindfulness practice.

☙ Mindful Moment: Neuropeptides

Candace Pert, PhD, author of *Molecules of Emotion: The Science Behind Mind-Body Medicine,* has famously stated that your body is your subconscious mind. Our physical body can be changed by the emotions we experience:

> Neuropeptides—molecules used by neurons to communicate with each other—carry emotional messages. As your feelings change, these biochemicals of emotion travel throughout your body and your brain, literally altering the chemistry of every cell in your body. A feeling sparked in our mind—or body—will translate as a peptide being released somewhere. [Organs, tissues, skin, muscle and endocrine glands]—they all have peptide receptors on them and can access and store emotional information. This means the emotional memory is stored in many places in the body, not just or even primarily, in the brain. You can access emotional memory anywhere in the peptide/receptor network, in any number of ways . . . unexpressed emotions are literally lodged in the body. The real true emotions that need to be expressed are in the body, trying to move up and be expressed and thereby integrated, made whole, and healed.[2]

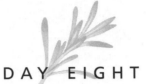

meditation on bodily sensations

If we are to wake up out of our patterning, a key element of that is to be able to pause, recognize, and open to a larger space than the cocoon that our mind is creating in thought. Our tendency is to get lost in a cycle of reactivity. In order to be able to step out of that cycle, we need to cultivate the ability to pause, recognize, and open.

—Tara Brach, Insight Meditation Teacher

MEDITATION PRACTICE: *8 minutes*

Day Eight, *Meditation on Bodily Sensations*

Mindfulness of the breath and body is the first critical step for learning how to regulate negative or repetitive thoughts. By training your attention to return, repeatedly, to the anchor of your breath, you start to develop the concentration essential for navigating and investigating bodily sensations. Meditation on bodily sensations further cultivates your awareness of the present-moment experience, making it a direct tool for working with feelings and thoughts. Changes in somatosensation—conscious perception of temperature, pressure, and vibration, introduced yester-day—grab your awareness in a unique way by shifting your attention in the process of "actively" sitting still. Sometimes these changing physical sensations are easier to detect than wanderings of thought.

Mindful awareness of bodily sensations can also be quite relaxing. It will help you both release tension and better understand its sources. Best of all, it teaches you how you can manage your thought patterns. This leads to greater equanimity and more skillful living by getting to the origins of your disquieting states—simply by observing the bodily sensations that teach you, in a new way, so much about your thoughts.

Investigating bodily sensations with kind attention can become your greatest ally in alleviating your own distress. Key to giving you insights into your reactions and thinking habits, meditation on bodily sensations helps you differentiate your direct experience from rumination, story lines, and automatic reaction. As you more clearly distinguish stress-inducing add-ons from direct experience—*presence*—you will begin to have more and more moments of relaxation, ease, and happiness.

Our bodies always give us signs about what is happening mentally and emotionally at any given moment. Yet in our typical busy and dis-tracted state, we are usually not attentive to them, thus missing an easily accessible, profound way to become more familiar with how mindful-ness works. Along with the more obvious attention grabbers—a knot in your shoulders, butterflies in your stomach—there is an entire world of more subtle physical phenomena present to inform you. By investigat-ing these physical sensations, you become aware of the point at which reaction begins—your window of opportunity to choose a different path of response.

So far your focus for meditation practice has been on the primary anchor: the breath. In today's lesson, you'll learn how to expand med-itative focus to a secondary anchor: bodily sensations. We'll start with expanding awareness from the breath to general awareness of the rest of the body.

Meditation on Bodily Sensations

Begin the meditation on bodily sensations in the same way as every mindfulness practice. That means position; anchor at the feeling of the breath; intention of time and attitude of kindness, equanimity, and patience; and remindfulness.

To get started, begin with a few minutes of meditation on the breath. As you attend to the sensations of the in-and-out of respiration, notice if you can detect any sensation on the area where the breath is entering your body in addition to the feel of the breath, at the area right beneath the nostrils. Then, expand your field of awareness beyond the breath anchor to include an awareness of the energies in the rest of your body. As you go more global, become aware of the sensations and feelings that tell you your body is alive. You may detect, for example, tingling in your hands or feet. You may experience some sensations you aren't otherwise aware of—accumulated tension in the shoulders, neck, or face. This may be because, other than the practice you have been doing with mindfulness of breath, you are not used to sitting still unless your attention is focused on some external phenomenon such as reading, working on a project, cooking, or watching a movie. These sensations have been there all along. You just haven't turned your attention to them in quite the same way.

Perhaps your body is completely at ease and relaxed. It's quite possible that you will experience a little bit of both pleasant and unpleasant sensations during this investigation. You are not seeking any one experience over another; you are simply attentive to whatever is presenting itself to you with curiosity and a willingness to be present.

Return your awareness to the physical sensations of the breath again. Now, with attention on the sensations of breathing in the foreground of your attention, if and when a physical sensation from some other part of your body commands your attention, simply move your awareness from the breath to the new predominant experience. This becomes your new anchor. With gentle attention and curiosity, observe these physical sensations. When your mind wanders—which it will—and you lose the mindful connection with the sensation, gently return your attention to the physical sensation. Keep the same attitude of nonjudgment that you have been cultivating in mindfulness of the breath meditation. Let go of any evaluation or commentary that may arise. Simply experience the physical sensations directly.

In relaxed fashion, explore the particular sensations that make it up—hardness or softness, warmth or coolness, tingling, tenseness, pressure, burning, itching, lightness, and so on. Notice what happens to the sensations as you are mindful of them. Do they become stronger or weaker, larger or smaller, or do they stay the same? Sense directly the experience and what happens to it as you are present for it.

Notice when the focus of your attention moves from the physical sensations to your reactions to the sensations and your thoughts about them or what may have been their cause. Do you want a certain sensation to go away? If this happens, simply move your attention back to the felt-sense of the sensations. Once a physical sensation is no longer compelling or has disappeared, return to mindfulness of breathing as your anchor until or if another sensation calls your attention.

As with all mindfulness meditation, you are simply practicing being present with whatever shows up. You attend to all the bodily sensations with the same attention and care as you have been practicing with mindfulness of the breath. When you open yourself to the experience of sensations in your body, they will reveal to you reactions, conflicts, or difficulties that have been stored as sensations in your body. As you hold these sensations in your awareness, they may change. They may dissolve and release. They may intensify, then vanish. They may remain for a while. It is not your job to try to do anything with them or push them away. Simply acknowledge them and be present. If at any time these sensations become overwhelming or too uncomfortable, simply return to your anchor point at the breath until you feel ready to open up to physical sensations as anchor once again.

Continue practicing mindfulness of bodily sensations in this fashion for the remainder of today's practice. If at any time you simply feel lost and unable to focus, bring your attention back to anchor at the breath. It's always a place to return to as primary anchor.

🪷 Mindful Moment: Back into Your Body

You may discover that you cannot detect any sensations in your body during today's meditation. If so, that's fine. This is perfectly normal and the experience of many people when just getting started with meditation on bodily sensations. It does not mean that these sensations are not there. This simply gives you more information about where you are in connecting mind with body. We are unaccustomed to paying attention to sensations that are usually just going on in the background while we are going about our daily activities. Your task is to open your awareness to anything that does arise. As you explore bodily sensations, when your mind wanders away, as soon as you notice it, gather your attention again at the breath anchor until you regain focus. Then open awareness again to the body as you feel ready.

If you are not aware of any physical sensations, you can recover this connection. A good place to start is to become aware of any contact points your body has with other objects. Can you feel your hips or the backs of your thighs on the chair? Can you feel your legs in contact with the surface beneath you? This, too, is physical sensation. As you deepen your awareness of the feeling of these contact points, you are practicing bringing conscious awareness to physical sensation. Soon, you will start to detect other sensations that are arising independent of contact points.

Through the meditation on bodily sensations, you become freshly aware of the physical connection to emotional states throughout the day. You might, for example, find yourself in the middle of a hectic afternoon, gripped with tightness in your shoulders that you may not have been aware of before—giving you a new opportunity to release tension before it becomes a mountain of unmanageable stress. Tomorrow, we'll progress from today's general awareness to a specific progressive strategy of meditation on bodily sensations.

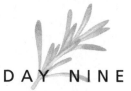

DAY NINE

body survey

*Meditation practice isn't about trying to throw ourselves away
and become something better. It's about befriending
who we are already.*

—PEMA CHÖDRÖN

MEDITATION PRACTICE: *9 minutes*

DAY NINE, *Body Survey I*

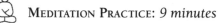 How was your experience of yesterday's meditation? Were you able to easily perceive sensations in your body? Perhaps no physical sensations captured your attention. Either way is perfectly fine. After all, we're just getting started with the mindfulness meditation process. And you've only had one day of practice at the meditation of bodily sensations. Which makes this the perfect time to introduce the body survey. This is a helpful tool for *reestablishing* the connection of brain to body.

Bettering the Mind-Body Connection

The body survey is a proven utensil for helping make the mindful connection with the sensations in your body. It is also a very healing and relaxing meditation on its own. It is a large and integral part of my daily formal meditation practice. It is also a process that I incorporate throughout the day in informal practice as an effective way of navigating the day's experiences.

With the body-survey meditation, you systematically move your attention through the body, noting any physical sensations you discover. The body survey can be practiced in any position. Start by gathering your attention via your established practice of mindfulness on the breath for a few minutes. Become keenly tuned in to the sensations right beneath the nose where the breath enters the body.

Then, bring this focused attention to the very top of your head. Rather than *picturing* this spot, *feel* whatever physical sensations you have in the area. It can be anything—a tingling, warmth, coolness, subtle vibration. Whatever sensations present themselves to you.

After feeling sensations at the top of your head, gently move down your face, observing the sensations through your forehead, eyebrows, eyelids, nose, cheeks, and lips—through the entire front of your head— to your chin. You will probably notice a tendency to visualize the body part you are focusing upon. Visualizing something means you are imagining, and you want to directly experience what *is*. If you notice yourself visualizing, simply return your attention to the actual physical sensations themselves. Repeat this scan from the top of your head through the back and sides of your head, so that your entire scalp has been scanned for physical sensations.

Once you have completed the scan of your head, progress to the front and back of your neck. Then, bring your attention up to the left shoulder. Survey the shoulder area, and then move attentive focus down every inch of your left arm, including the front and back of the upper arm, the elbow, the forearm, and every inch of your hand including the back of your hand, the palm, and the fingers. Next, complete the same investigation of the right arm, starting at the right shoulder, surveying the right upper arm in front and back, the elbow, the forearm. Bring your attention to the back of the right hand, the palm, and every finger on your right hand. What sensations do you feel? Is there tingling, throbbing, itching—perhaps even awareness of your pulse? Other sensations might be warmth or coolness, vibration, and/or numbness.

If at any point in time your mind wanders from the body scan, as soon as you are aware of it, bring your mind back to the point of concentration on today's anchor, mindfulness of bodily sensation, and pick up where you left off, just as you would in mindfulness of breath. You can implement mental noting by quietly saying "Thinking" in the background to help bring you gently back to anchor. If you detect a sensation that's uncomfortable, you might reflexively try to push it away or feel anger or fear. If you experience any such reactions, note them, and see if you can release them equanimously, and bring your attention back to the direct experience of the moment. What is the actual sensation of the discomfort—or pleasure? Feel it directly, without judgment or mental interpretation. Emotions such as impatience, enjoyment, boredom, joy, or sadness might arise as well. Acknowledge everything with patience, and return gently to the body scan. Cultivating equanimity in the face of the changing experience of bodily sensations translated directly to equanimity in your daily life.

During the survey, you might also come across patches—even entire areas of your body—where you can perceive no physical sensations. Simply note these blind spots as you do each sensation. With continued practice, the sensations of these areas will come more into your awareness. All in its own good time.

Move on to your collarbone, noting the sensations across the entire expanse. Zigzag gently down the front of your chest and torso, noting any sensations from your armpits, your sides, and all the way down to your waist and below, into the front of your pelvis and into the pelvic floor.

If you find it difficult to stay with bodily sensation at all, then simply return to your primary anchor, the breath, until you can recover focus and a degree of concentration. Then, return to the body survey at the point at which you left off.

Next, bring your attention to the top of the back, and survey for bodily sensations all the way down your back, meandering from one side to the other, being attentive to every space in two- or three-inch increments, all the way down to the bottom of the back. Let your attention to sensation continue to the lower back, then to the hips. Investigate the sensations throughout the back of your hips, all the way from one side to another.

Continue the body survey down your legs. With curiosity, investigate the sensations starting at the top and front of your left thigh, sweeping down toward the knee. Note any sensations in your left knee; then continue down through the left shin to your ankle, to the top of your foot, and all the way down to each toe on the left foot. Let your attention then move over the toes to the bottom of the left foot, to the heel, to the back of the ankle, and then up the back of the left leg. Feel the sensations in the left calf, in the back of the knee, and all the way up the back of the left thigh to your hip. Move your attention to the front of the right leg at the hip, and continue the scan on your right leg, scanning the top of the thigh to the knee and down the shin of the right leg. Feel any sensations on your right ankle, on the top of the foot, through every toe on your right foot, and on to the bottom of your right foot. Note any tingling, warmth, coolness, itching—any of it.

Continue up the back of the right ankle, surveying the sensations up the back of the right leg through the calf, to the back of the knee, and all the way up the back of the right thigh to your hip. Each time your mind starts to wander to thought, planning, or remembering, or brings the urge to move, simply return to the point of the body scan that you last remember, and continue. You can always return to the anchor at the breath to gain more stability of concentration. Should you discover that you absolutely must move, mindfully adjust your position and come back to meditation.

Depending on time constraints or the situation in which you find yourself, you can do a quick body survey in mere seconds as a technique to ground yourself and bring yourself into the present. Each time you direct your attention to physical sensation as you do with the body survey, you reinforce the connection of body, mind, and emotion. After all, it is about being in touch with the whole of your being—including your body—in any and every way you can. You can practice body surveys, whether brief or lengthy, lying in bed in the morning before you get up or at night before you go to sleep. You can also practice them sitting or standing—in any situation.

🪷 Mindful Moment: The STOP Strategy

Checking in with your mind and body during the day increases your awareness of physical sensations and patterns of thinking, helping you become more connected to yourself, aware of reactivity, and allowing you to self-regulate emotion, and thought, and increase your sense of well-being.

STOP, an acronym for a process often used in mindfulness training, gives you a tool for quickly checking in with mental activity and bodily sensation. It is a proven avenue for helping you be more mindful throughout the day. A convenient tool for leveraging you out of the default mode network and its potential for accelerating anxiety, rumination, and inner combat, STOP works as follows:

S	**Stop.** Whatever you are doing at the moment, pause. If you can't actually stop what you are doing—pushing your cart through the line at the market, for example—simply put the pause button on the activities of your mind.
T	**Take a breath.** Be attentive to the sensation of the breath as it enters and exits your body. Recalling and feeling your meditation anchor point at this time instantly connects your formal practice with this informal practice.
O	**Observe what is happening for you in this very moment.** What is going on in your mind? Are you agitated, hurried, or worried? Are you juggling a million projects in your head? Are you excited, happy, or calm? Turning your attention to your body, what can you bring into your awareness? Can you sense your posture, any sensations? Tension or relaxation? Check in with everything—breath, body, and mind. Simply investigate, without designs to push away or suppress any experience.
P	**Proceed.** Move forward with your day.

STOP is easy and quick to implement, no matter how pressed you are for time. With practice, you will be able to squeeze in a quick STOP in five seconds—anywhere, any time.

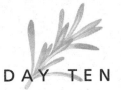

kathryn—from food free fall to eating freedom

It is never too late to turn on the light. Your ability to break an unhealthy habit or turn off an old tape doesn't depend on how long it has been running... When you flip the switch in that attic, it doesn't matter whether it's been dark for ten minutes, ten years or ten decades. The light still illuminates the room and banishes the murkiness.

—Sharon Salzberg, *Real Happiness: The Power of Meditation*

Meditation Practice: *10 minutes*

Day Ten, *Body Survey II*

The skills of awareness and thought management you are practicing translate directly to the eating experience. Here's a powerful example to illustrate.

Making the Connection: Kathryn's Story

Kathryn was two weeks into mindfulness practice when we had our third coaching session. She had been doing formal meditations for ten to fifteen minutes daily for two weeks.

One of Kathryn's biggest challenges—a pattern of falling away every seven to ten days from her aspirations to eat plant-based whole food—had not materialized since she had begun her daily meditations.

"Mindfulness meditation has been easier to follow. It is easier for me to get focused, not go with thoughts as they come up, and return to attention on the breath. I am also more interested in doing exercise," Kathryn said. She shared that she was feeling a lot better, had a lot more energy, and was down three pounds.

I asked Kathryn to tell me more about "feeling better" and "more energy." How did that show up for her?

Kathryn's Backstory

When Kathryn first contacted me, she had been trying to eat a healthier plant-based diet for about four years. A busy nursing professor, she had also experienced during those four years deep stress with the loss of three close family members. And her daughter was about to give birth to Kathryn's next grandchild.

While pleased with the results she had experienced to date with her plant-based eating, including a ten-pound weight loss, Kathryn felt stalled in her progress.

"I haven't been eating as well," she told me. "I am feeling lousy—like I am in a hole." She found herself in a disheartening loop of getting stricter with her diet, going along fine for about a week, and then it would all "fall apart."

I asked Kathryn to tell me more about her struggle. In addition to the seven-to-ten-day "fallout" phenomenon, every afternoon, between two and four o'clock, she would start to crave pretzels—handily available in the vending machine down the hall. The craving wouldn't let go until she went down the hall, bought the pretzels, and ate them. Sometimes multiple bags.

To complicate matters, Kathryn had been trying to implement a strictly structured plant-based dietary plan that was focused on weight loss. This regimen required eliminating many wholesome plant foods, such as nuts. It demanded that she scrupulously police any speck of processed foods in her diet and that she eat certain foods at certain times of the day. Lots of rules.

Kathryn had started to feel that if she wasn't doing this plan 100 percent, then she just wasn't doing well at all. She would be able to stick with this strict plan for about a week, at which point she would be unable to continue, and the whole plan would crumble. Then, once she mustered her energy for another go, she would start again. Seven to ten days seemed to be, historically, Kathryn's breaking point.

"I want to be happy and have more joy in my life!" Kathryn told me. She also wanted to lose about twenty pounds. While firmly committed to plant-based eating, she was getting the sense that just steeling herself for another round of a highly regimented food plan was not the answer for her. Kathryn was looking for something different.

Two-Week Report

As Kathryn continued to tell me about the past week, she happily reported that the seven-to-ten-day fallout had not materialized. This she attributed to a couple of things. First, she had realized during our initial conversation that getting stricter with her plant-based diet was not what she needed. Softening her approach to eating from the strict plan, while still eating predominantly whole plant foods, helped. The strict approach, Kathryn said, "is not a good fit for me," since it simply added to her anxiety around eating and her overall stress. Second, she realized that her daily mindfulness meditation practice was making her more conscious of her thought patterns and reactions during the day—the first step toward changing them.

I asked Kathryn if the recurring pretzel predicament had presented itself this week.

"Yesterday," Kathryn continued, "by four o'clock I started to crave the pretzels." Here is where her mindfulness meditation practice, Kathryn said, made all the difference between this day turning into a "fallout"—and the fact that it didn't.

Eating Freedom

To get more information about what might have inspired the late-afternoon desire for the quick, crunchy comfort that the pretzels would provide, I asked Kathryn if she was, perhaps, simply hungry. Kathryn said that hunger was not the issue. She had eaten a hearty whole-grain breakfast and a robust salad at lunch. She had been taking to heart my suggestion to eat several servings of beans every day. Eliminating hunger as the pull to eat is important so that we can respond skillfully to the moment. When you're hungry, the skillful response is to eat. With hunger off the table, we are invited to look further.

It's important to get one thing straight. Though not an exemplary-quality whole plant food, the pretzels themselves are not the bugbear here. There's nothing wrong with eating a few pretzels now and then. It is the situation around them and the change in behavior that they represented for Kathryn that was the problem. This freedom to make new choices as Kathryn has done is real.

Every time you become aware of a thought, rather than lost in a thought, you experience an opening of the mind and heart. The opening to new possibility. The whole question of our bondage or freedom—with food or anything else for that matter—hinges on what choices we make with respect to those thoughts. Through a mindfulness meditation practice, you become skilled in this awareness of thought and opportunity to new choices—which, as Kathryn demonstrates, is directly applicable to eating.

Previously, in response to the pretzel urge, Kathryn had done her darndest to dredge up willpower, which never seemed to have a fighting chance. Before, she would have engaged in the pretzel war in her mind: they weren't good for her diet, they would throw her off track, why did she want them anyway since she wasn't hungry, and on and on. The pretzels would haunt her until she caved. Which she did. Every time.

This time, Kathryn told me, the process was entirely different. She had the presence of mind to respond skillfully. She approached the desire for pretzels as she does thoughts during meditation—as an interested, curious, nonjudgmental observer. In contrast to her old method of immediately diving into the pretzels, or simply holding off long enough until the inevitable took place, she was able to see, first of all, that the thought of the pretzels was just that. A *thought*. A thought with a strong pull, for sure.

Yet because she had been practicing mindful awareness of thoughts and the bodily sensations connected to them during her two weeks of meditations—*what you practice grows stronger*—she was able to observe the desire to reach for the pretzels as it showed up as thoughts in her mind and as tension in her body. Within a few minutes of its onset, the urge for the pretzels dissolved, and Kathryn went about her day— without giving the pretzels another thought. She recognized that her previous, conditioned response to the pretzels—desire, followed by debate, followed by indulgence, followed by remorse—was a habit pattern, rife with judgment and confusion.

Kathryn had faced the underlying tension that was presenting itself in the form of the pretzel urge. She allowed herself to be present with the discomfort directly, rather than by reacting with an eating behavior that was incompatible with her goals of health and restoring an inner balance. Instead of getting lost in the debate or mental negotiations, which can suck her right into the default mode network where cravings also reside, she made a more skillful choice to stay mindful of what was happening.

Most importantly, she had a newfound freedom to make that choice. Choosing in this way has started to loosen the tethers to the pretzels. She is setting a new behavior pattern of being present and mindful and moving unscathed right through the middle of it all. She has increased real ease around the eating experience by discerning stress eating from mindful eating.

This is precisely where mindfulness delivers such strength and freedom. Mindfulness allows the possibility of not reacting habitually or blindly on the energy of uninvited thoughts.

Rather, it helps you choose wisely. Even if we have chosen unwisely in the past, in the moment of awakening to the possibilities of mindfulness and skillful action, a shift takes place.

As you go through the day, note any thoughts or urges that arise similar to the pretzel urge that Kathryn experienced. There may be certain times during the day that you can think of right now when the pull to diffuse tension or other discomfort by urging you to put something in your mouth presents itself. It could be another behavior that has become a problematic diversion. Next time one of these situations comes up—where you feel compelled by something other than hunger to grab an edible, for example—note the thought. It will no doubt be very compelling to you—as if once the thought occurs, follow-through is a given. After all, that's what you've probably done over and over again. And it may be thus next time, too. Yet awareness of this thought, and recognition that it is just a thought, is an important development in your ability to act more mindfully when such situations arise. As soon as possible, observe the thought—whether pretzel or otherwise—as a thought. Without suppressing it, or fighting it, or ignoring it, let your attention shift from the "pretzels" themselves to the phenomenon of the thought and the feelings in your body that come along with it.

☙ Mindful Moment: Bundled Behaviors

Perhaps you have experienced something similar to Kathryn. A "munchies" habit that you've found recurs in a certain place, or time, or both—and that you've found impossible to shake. As I explained to Kathryn, behaviors that we are desirous of changing, such as reaching for the pretzels, are often parts of a bundle. A package of habituated responses from our past that have created the conditions for the present. Unpacking Kathryn's pretzel "package" revealed several components: her busy teaching schedule, responsibilities with students, and family commitments all had converged at the "appointed" hour, thus driving the compelling pretzel scenario. Yet there's even more complexity to the bundle. With a mountain of work to do at her desk, Kathryn was also in a particular place (her office at work) at a particular time (four o'clock) that for her have historically been associated with eating pretzels. That's a lot of pieces to the package coming together at once. The pull of past practices can suck us in before we even know what hit us. We can find ourselves halfway through the bag of pretzels before we even come up for air. And by then we have usually tainted the whole affair with guilt, remorse, and anxiety so much that we aren't really enjoying the pretzels anyway.

This time, Kathryn was able to do something different. Drawing upon her mindfulness meditation practice, she was able to approach the situation—the crisis point with the pretzels—in a new fashion: as being compelled by past practices and conditioning. Watching the situation, the behavior bundle, around the pretzel pattern unfold was also enlightening. Kathryn's daily mindfulness meditation practice made it possible for her to unravel this established behavior bundle. Her daily practice had paid off in a significant way. By responding with mindfulness as she did, Kathryn has set a new precedent. It will make this response even easier to implement at future incidents should they arise, because she has created a new set of skills.

Every day we live out, and act out, all our old, conditioned—due to repetition—habit patterns. It is deeply difficult to step outside these patterns in a way that allows us to see these habits of reaction, whether in thought or deed, and see them for what they are—conditioned responses often presented in behavior bundles. With mindfulness practice, by gaining some new perspectives on these bundles in a way that allows us to discern what is actually happening and find a fresh way, we can make new, skillful choices based on wisdom rather than reactive conditioning.

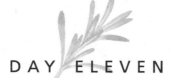

hindrances, antidotes, and helping factors

Mindfulness is about paying attention to our present moment experiences, with openness and curiosity, and a willingness to be with what is.

—DIANA WINSTON, Director of Mindfulness Education, UCLA Mindful Awareness Research Center

MEDITATION PRACTICE: *11 minutes*

DAY ELEVEN, *Hindrances and Helping Factors*

In the longtime tradition of mindfulness meditation, going back thousands of years, a handful of obstacles have emerged as common hindrances to meditation practice. From time to time, all of us will be troubled by one or the other of them. Having an awareness of them early on can help shape your practice for the better. Looking directly at these hindrances, should they be in your experience, allows them to be your greatest teachers. Through meditation practice you are cultivating a stable, clear awareness that bolsters your inner resources to meet these impediments, detailed below. I've included antidotes to help and added some bonus tips for mindfulness practice as well.

The Five Classic Hindrances to Mindfulness Practice

These are five common challenges to meditation practice—and tried and true antidotes to skillfully manage them. I've added applications for informal practice "off the meditation cushion."

Restlessness

Do you ever find that after sitting in meditation practice for a few minutes—or even sooner—you become restless, perhaps a bit bored, and have the urge to jump out of your seat and start on with your other projects for the day? This should not be surprising. After all, it is our lifelong habit to go, achieve, and get on to the next thing. We're trained from a very young age to do, do, and then do some more. Our culture, the media, even our technology reinforce a frenetic pace, urging us to acquire, consume, produce, and move at an ever faster pace. Is it any wonder our minds don't take quickly to simply being?

Restlessness takes many forms. Racing mind. Physical agitation. The urge to get up. Adjusting your position. Scratching an itch. Obsessive planning—of your life, an upcoming vacation, a project at work, or dinner. Or you might feel bored. As our minds are used to having their way with our attention, taking us all over the place with stories or other exciting activities, to simply not play along in the usual fashion might seem like something of a letdown. Where's the excitement?

Antidote: Although we tend to think of restlessness as physical, it is a manifestation of mental restlessness. Restlessness and boredom are merely thoughts and sensations. Which means they can be treated like any other thought or sensation. If you look closely at restlessness or boredom, often underneath them you will find some measure of anxiety or other emotional unsettlement. Simply recognizing restlessness in one of its many guises can help lessen its influence. When restlessness or boredom arise, use them as objects of your meditation by noticing how they show up as sensations in your body accompanied by thoughts—a long list of reasons to think about or go do something else. Yes, boredom is a thought and has a "feeling" to it. A quick body survey (page 81) can help you find these sensations of restlessness if they aren't immediately apparent to you. This way, you deal with the state of restlessness directly—a tremendously useful tool for on the meditation cushion and off.

One of the important reasons for sitting in formal practice for progressively longer periods is because the skill of navigating restlessness during practice time is pivotal to mindfully navigating thoughts, emotions, and experiences outside of formal practice. If every time you feel an itch you scratch it, or every two minutes you adjust your position or follow the urge to plan that inspired and brilliant project, you are reinforcing the neurological pathway to latch onto an impulse and let it take you on its compelling ride. With mindfulness training, instead of trying to muster up willpower and not do something, you stay present with the thought, emotion, or experience as it arises—attentively aware of it, curiously noting its presence, without rejecting its presence or identifying with it. Big difference.

Tips for Informal Practice: Working with restlessness during formal meditation practice will make you more attuned to states of restlessness and her various incarnations that emerge at other times during your day. Normally, we get caught up in the push and pull of our daily experience. The know-how you acquire during formal practice is directly transferable to these moments. Unsettled states or agitation will be more quickly recognized as they arise. By building the neurological pathways of patience and observation, you will be able to increasingly draw on these skills outside of formal practice. The direct result is better choices, more skillful living, greater equanimity, and patience—another reason you practice patience for yourself *during* formal practice. How we relate to our feelings and thoughts makes all the difference.

No matter where you are, when restlessness or boredom come up, you can quickly do a body survey. The process of RAIN (page 134) is also a perfect match. You now have a practiced protocol for moving through restlessness in a way that doesn't act it out, deny it, or bury it for later.

Wanting/Desire/Craving

Seemingly related to restlessness, wanting, desire, and craving are in a hindrance category of their own. You may notice that as soon as you sit down to meditation, you want to be somewhere else. Or you start to think, wouldn't a bite to eat be nice? and your thoughts are off and running with different food topics. Perhaps wanting shows up as the desire for conditions to be different. If only it were warmer, you think. Or cooler. Or my cushion were softer. These thoughts can ignite restlessness, looping you back to hindrance number one.

Of course, wanting and desire are thoughts and feelings that arise a million times a day outside of formal practice. Let's have this for a snack, let's get a new car, let's remodel the kitchen... These desires are not bad in themselves, of course. Yet once you start being mindful of your states of mind, you start to see how often our inner peace is subject to the pull of yet another wanting, desiring, or craving.

Antidote: Desire comes with a companion: the underlying illusion that we can actually find satisfaction by acquiring every thing or experience we crave. The irony is that craving and desire only create more craving and desire. This doesn't mean that you should never follow through on acquiring something you want or need. At the same time, developing the skill during formal meditation to see this runaway train of desires and wants as objects is valuable practice for more discriminating thought through the rest of the day.

If the mind is busy wanting to be somewhere else during your meditation practice, you can use it as an object of your meditation. What does this desire and wanting feel like in your body? Simply continue to notice the thoughts straying and gently, patiently bring your attention back to anchor every time you notice it has wandered. If it continues to be a strong pull, shift to another meditation strategy that might keep things more interesting for your mind while still staying present, such as mindfulness of bodily sensations. This can be another good time to implement the body survey.

Tips for Informal Practice: If you think about it, most of our moments are driven by the desire to get something we want, hang on to or avoid losing something we have—whether an object or an experience—or to get something other than what we are currently experiencing, if our current experience is not to our liking. Seeking pleasure and avoiding pain shape our lives and are not inherently bad. Most desires are harmless and actually necessary: the desire to eat when hungry, cover up when cold, and get out of the lightning storm. Yet they can also have an insidious way of trying to run the show, with little regard for our happiness. Allure can quickly lead to regret, impulsivity to unfavorable outcomes, and reactivity to remorse. Mindfulness practice develops your strength of discrimination. By learning to be patiently present with the rising of desire and the wanting of this and that during formal practice, you discover you can navigate these same thoughts and sensations that arise in the rest of your day. This translates directly into navigating urges to overeat, get carried away in a self-righteous argument, react angrily to getting cut off in traffic, check your Twitter feed—the applications are endless. You start with the small stuff, and don't be surprised when the bigger stuff gets easier. The practice of mindfully investigating and letting go of the little compulsions to scratch an itch during formal practice, adjust your cushion for the umpteenth time, or get up and move about transfers directly to having one cookie instead of ten. Instead of rolling your eyes and exploding in self-righteous indignation when one more person tells you they couldn't live without meat, you respond more skillfully. Reactivity can deepen problems—mindful presence opens insights into a better response.

So when desire arises, drop your attention into your body and investigate. What does this desire and wanting feel like in your body? Is it a signal your body is sending to do something important—such as eat a meal or take a nap—or is it the fallout from reactivity? With practice, your discriminatory powers will become clearer.

Resistance

Call it irritation or aversion, this hindrance has many faces and can show up as depression, hatred, or even anger. Maybe we don't feel like we're having a good meditation experience. Maybe something seems to be disturbing our attempt to meditate, such as noise in the room. Or maybe resistance has arrived as a secondary emotion, right on the heels of restlessness. We're resisting the experience as it is. Or we're irritated that we're so restless!

Antidote: It's at times like these that I like to call on the words of one of my teachers, Diana Winston, also the epigraph of this chapter: "Mindfulness is about paying attention to our present moment experiences, with openness and curiosity, and a willingness to be with what is." Oh yeah, that's right! It's not about seeking any particular experience, or embracing one and pushing away another—the practice is fundamentally returning your attentive awareness to whatever is coming up in the moment, without judgment. Simply bringing this to mind is usually enough to snap me out of the resistant state.

Tips for Informal Practice: Developing the skill to be present with irritation, resistance, and things you don't like puts you back in control by relinquishing it. When you feel resistance, anger, or irritation, it can be very natural to justify your experience, and before you know it, you are caught up in the story. That rude offhanded remark by a coworker? I'll show them! The insensitive comment by your spouse? How dare they! Get cut off in traffic by a road-raged driver? Who do they think they are? Resistance can be addressed by looking directly to the feelings that are arising in your body. Tension in the abdomen; tightness in the face. The effect is that, instead of being caught up in the drama and accelerating the collateral damage, you restore a sense of groundedness. This has the effect of keeping you more even-minded so that you can respond more skillfully. If you have been wronged and need to speak up, this approach will give you a better chance at being more calm and clear in delivery, while also helping you shake a painful compulsion to be "right." The more you practice this skill, grounded in your mindfulness practice, the better you get at it and the easier it comes.

Sleepiness

Being sleep deprived as many of us are, is it any wonder that when we take a step away from our active lives and swirling minds that we want to nod off? Another reason sleepiness might hit when we sit down to meditate is because we are feeling overwhelmed by the experience, or something is uncomfortable about the meditation that day—either physically, mentally, or emotionally—and we'd rather just check out. Sleep allows us to back away from the discomfort.

Antidote: Perhaps your posture is too slumpy, or you collapsed your position without knowing it, detracting from an energetic and focused posture. Gently, and with mindfulness, you can reestablish position and bring yourself to a greater state of alertness. Another idea is to stand up for a few minutes, as you can meditate standing up. If you meditate in the morning and find sleepiness is a frequent visitor, you can splash water on your face before getting started. I always turn on the lights in the room for a couple of minutes before I sit down for practice—as soon as the bright light hits the eyes, there is an awakening effect. And finally, if during an occasional sitting you find yourself drifting off into sleep over and over again, you probably just need a good nap. So take it!

Tips for Informal Practice: Recurring sleepiness during your meditation practice may be a sign that you aren't getting enough sleep. There are all kinds of suggestions available for what to do to secure your required hours—dark room and no thriller novels or movies at bedtime, to name a couple. Rather than list them all here, because I think these are different for everybody, find out what seems to have bearing on your sleep time, and take steps as needed.

Doubt

Indecision. Skepticism. Uncertainty about whether or not this will work. Doubt can be a healthy thing while we are making an initial evaluation about whether to buy or try anything. Yet if we keep digging up the seed to see if it's sprouting, we interrupt an important process. Too much doubt too soon can pull us away from an experience before we even give it a chance.

Antidote: First, remember that thoughts are just thoughts, and may or may not be facts. Just because you think it, it doesn't make it true. When you detect doubt slipping in during your formal practice, note it just as any other thought. You may well be able to detect an accompanying emotion or sensation underneath it—sadness or restlessness, for example. This gives you specific material for your meditation because you can detect it as a bodily sensation.

Tips for Informal Practice: Setting doubt aside during your formal practice time does not mean that you should not evaluate the pros and cons of meditation or anything else. During meditation practice, however, is not the time. It's just another way for your active, roving mind to go off task. Rather, make the decision to address any doubts later on, outside of meditation time.

❧ Mindful Moment: Helping Factors

The attitude you bring to your practice is important for creating an atmosphere conducive to developing mindfulness. It has tremendous bearing on awakening the skills—and rewards—of mindfulness practice.

- **Be kind and gentle**. Foster a spirit of kindness and compassion toward yourself. Rather than thinking about formal mindfulness practice as another "should" to add to your to-do list, cultivate an attitude of choosing to practice because you care about clarity and inner peace. Let this be the atmosphere that nurtures your practice. I've listed this helping factor first because it colors everything about your meditation experience and informal practice, and it is reflected in who you are in the world. More about this on Day Twenty (page 162).
- **Take your time**. When you sit for formal practice, invest the few seconds it takes to be relaxed and at ease yet attentive in your body. Let go of the urge to rush. Patience and acceptance are the watchwords here. Meditation may at times be hard work, but it is not a combat zone. Remember that it is remindfulness and not a perfectly still mind that is important, so take the time you need to settle in.
- **Enjoy the journey**. While our minds like to get all revved up and distracted with expectations, this attitude is itself a tendency of the mind. Mindfulness practice asks that we suspend preconceptions and ideas in preference for what *is*. Relax, follow the simple instructions to the best of your ability, and watch the effects show up in your life. Don't be surprised if, right next to the usual distractions and agitations, you find insights, connections, and expansive moments of joy and happiness rise unexpectedly during the day.

- **Problem-solve later.** You may find that inspiration for good ideas, insights into solving problems, or excitement about one project or another arises during your meditation. It may seem like a good time to go ahead and let your mind invest the energy and figure something out. It may feel irresistible, in fact! Yet now is not the time to ponder. Discursive reasoning and talks with yourself are best put aside until after formal practice. After all, now is the time for sharpening your tools of attentive awareness so that you can more skillfully wield them outside of formal practice.

- **Reconnect with your why.** What are your reasons for wanting to practice focusing your attention? Is it to increase self-regulation of emotions and reactions? To help regulate your nervous system and reduce stress? To explore what is going on in your inner landscape, so that you can know yourself better and find out what is driving your outer behavior? To gain freedom from the constant barrage of thoughts and mental activity? To have more equanimity in the face of the omnivorous spread at the company barbecue? To get mindless snacking off your back instead of trying to rearrange all the possible encounters you may have with tempting edibles? You now have a much stronger tool than hoping you don't get presented with hard-to-resists or hiding from them.

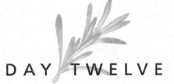

DAY TWELVE

big diet, binges, and a better way

The significant problems we face cannot be solved at the same level of thinking we were at when we created them.

—ALBERT EINSTEIN

🧘 MEDITATION PRACTICE: *12 minutes*

🔊 DAY TWELVE, *Meditation on Breath and Bodily Sensations*

💡 Mindless snacking, compulsive eating, overeating, bingeing—these are some of the painful problems reported by eaters everywhere. Often, they are accompanied by a weight struggle. Odds are that if you are plagued by challenges around food, weight is or has been an issue for you—whether you are truly "overweight" or not.

Yet there are exceptions. Even people who are not experiencing a struggle with poundage can be bedeviled by mindless snacking, transition eating, or an obsession with food, eating, or their weight. Either way, the diet industry is all too eager to hook us up with one weight-loss regimen or another.

There is good news from the research on how mindfulness can deliver us from the pain of eating problems. This includes one of the most troubling of eating behaviors: binge eating. Today we'll look at new insights into the diet industry and important research on relief—via mindfulness practice—from debilitating challenges, such as binge eating and related behaviors around food.

Big Diet

Big Diet hooks our desire to lose twenty pounds yesterday by convincing us that the solution to out-of-control eating is to tighten our grip on eating in hypercontrolled fashion. If we would only eat certain foods, at certain times, in certain amounts, we'll get control over our eating, get thin, and win the happiness it promises.

There's a palpable appeal to this authoritarian approach. If you're in pain, struggling to control your eating, or feeling shame about your size, it can feel like a huge relief to surrender to an outside authority that is telling you exactly what and when to eat and not eat. Yet not unlike the Chinese finger-trap toy—the harder you pull, the more your finger is stuck—clamping down with tighter control and rigidity on your eating always backfires. Sooner or later you're buried even deeper in the quicksand.

My most painful memory of a disastrous dalliance, decades ago, with a popular supervised diet program comes to mind. Desperate for help with my eating and weight after years of "failing" on my own, I braved the daunting territory of getting help by signing up for a diet program in town. As a health and fitness professional, asking for help was a tough move for me to make. But I swallowed my pride and made an appointment.

As soon as I sat down for the induction session with my diet "counselor," red flags started waving. The first question she asked me was, "What do you want to weigh?" I pulled my fantasy weight out of my hat—a number I hadn't seen since ninth grade. She wrote it down on my chart without question. So much for "counseling."

She proceeded to outline the specifics for my (at the time) vegetarian diet: one fruit a day, no "carbs" except for two whole-grain crackers, no sugar, lots of protein (tofu, tofu, and more tofu, as eggs were off my plate), and no beans or dairy products since they were too high in "carbs." I was required to weigh in at the center daily. Apparently, keeping me tethered to authority was critical.

What happened next should have had me running from the center as if from a burning building. Though I may not have qualified for an official binge eating disorder,[1] I could pound down the eats with the best of them. The problem was painful enough to drive me to talk to her about it. I broke down in tears, telling the counselor that I couldn't understand why—happily married and purposefully employed—I was driving around compulsively eating giant chocolate bars. She couldn't have gotten out of the room faster if an alien had popped out of the side of my head. So much for "counseling."

In spite of my better judgment and hooked by the relief it promised from my angst, I dove into the diet anyway. Eating strictly according to plan, I got within six pounds of my "goal" until my white knuckles of hunger gave out. I maintained my weight loss for precisely four hours before I dove into a stash of Christmas cookies. I put all the weight back on and more within weeks. In my zeal to achieve a fantasy weight, I'd forgotten, yet again, how undereating is always followed by overeating.

Doomed: The Weight-Centric Authoritarian Approach

Despite their rescue appeal, authoritarian approaches to eating, such as my experience with the diet program, set you up for problems. First, after exploiting our addiction to the next weight-loss magic bullet, the focus on weight loss and the strict controls over food to achieve it can hook your survival instinct by driving up hunger. Second, the obsessive thinking and extensive mental energy these plans demand can spiral you into negative mood states, sadness, and depression—let's not forget the lessons about the default mode network. Maintaining a focus on weight as the keystone for happiness elicits shame and remorse about your weight and errant eating. As alluring as prescriptive food plans may be due to the illusion of control, they barely give lip service to why we are overeating or eating the wrong foods in the first place. Despite what you may have heard, it's not just the food.

The research tells us that approaching weight issues in this fashion—with the main focus on weight loss itself, clinically known as a weight-centric approach—leads to high rates of weight regain, overall weight gain, adverse health, and diminished well-being. Long-term success at finding and maintaining your "goal weight" are doomed. People who try to achieve and maintain weight loss via regimented approaches are also at increased risk for eating disorders, disturbed eating behaviors, and a troubled relationship with their bodies. The dietary rigidity needed to maintain the weight loss, the shaming overtones of the programs themselves, and the binge eating that may follow once the diet is "broken" all play a part.[2]

The Behavioral Approach

Up until now, the treatment of choice for weight management under the weight-centric model has been what is known as the behavioral approach. With this method, the focus is one or another method of eat-less-move-more. Strict meal plans and tight rules around eating. Sound familiar? How'd that work for you, long term? The rules are some variation of the following: 1) avoid having temptation in the house or letting yourself anywhere near "trigger" foods or any place where you might encounter them; 2) get your mind off cravings by doing something to distract yourself when they come up; 3) reduce stress; and 4) get support.

If you have struggled with food and your weight, you don't need me to tell you that the behavioral method has delivered disappointing results. Even the research shows that while some people are successful at losing a fair amount of weight with this approach, most lose very little, and many—perhaps you know the feeling—even gain.[3] Most of the people who do lose weight in these programs put it all back on (plus more) in three to five years. We've heard this before. But we're never offered anything as a solution other than a stab at changing habits, platitudes like "Diets don't work," vague comments like "It's a lifestyle issue," or some other cliché designed to distract us from the fact that even the weight-loss experts are at a loss with what to do and hope we won't notice. Visions of my diet "counselor" come to mind. We're left with shattered hopes and aching hearts, without a clue as to how to make it all work, keeping our fingers crossed that we'll do better next time. Even then, we're haunted by the gnawing pain surrounding what we suspect by now is the main issue—our relationship with food, our bodies, our lives, or all of it.

It's not surprising that those who do better with the behavioral approach have done so because of ongoing close ties with a behavior counselor—kind of like a lifelong cheerleader.[4] Without changing the inner landscape, you'll most likely need someone to help you keep up the motivation and rely on the accountability/shame/fear factor to keep the whole weight-management machine going.

Even when accompanied by methods of behavior modification, weight-centric approaches skirt the issue by not addressing the heart of the problem. By fostering a preoccupation with your weight, they fail to help you with the internal issues that can fire up cravings and drive you to eat in ways that are inappropriate to your hunger and sense of fullness.[5] Which begs the question: Why spin your wheels pruning and trellising the branches of the problem when you can neutralize them at their roots—with mindfulness?

Going to the Roots of Dietary Disinhibition

People who report high levels of "internal disinhibition"—which means you are pretty good at rationalizing around and breaking the rules you've established for your diet—have a tendency to eat out of reactivity to their thoughts and feelings.[6] You may already know this about yourself. But what kind of practical guidance have you been given to change it?

If, up until now, you have been focused primarily on weight loss as the ticket to your well-being, happiness, freedom, and peace of mind—your success hinging on achieving a desired size—statistically, you will never either reach or sustain your goal. And let's be honest. Though you may have been telling yourself that your weight is not a contingency for you to feel happy, if you have been avoiding situations, places, or people or delaying anything at all until you get some weight off, then, in reality, you have.

Instead of policing yourself with meticulous food diaries, negative self-talk, bargaining your way out of a treat, or other tools of shame, if you are attentive to what makes you feel and function better in your everyday life, emotionally and physically, the outcomes can be radically different. Do you operate better when you eat more fruits and vegetables, drink more water, take a walk with a friend, meditate to relieve stress and to learn to self-regulate emotion, and get enough sleep? Have you ever experienced the way that an obsession with food falls away when you stop ignoring or suppressing your hunger signals? Now we're getting somewhere.[7]

As for the Last Few Pounds

A review of available advice for shaving off the "last five" (or ten) pounds delivers the usual disheartening results. On the up side are the references to increasing whole plant foods and eliminating fiber-free animal products. Yet more often we are urged to submit to a yearning to be thin by fasting, drawing bright lines around dessert, manipulating calorie intake up and down to "boost metabolism," or to other external methods of tightening control over what you eat. Rigid dieting is usually disrupted by episodes of overeating and is associated with eating in the absence of hunger, followed by attempts to compensate for calories consumed with excessive exercise, fasting, and the mental and emotional suffering that accompany them. It's only when you dig deep into the research that you find some real answers that don't exploit our peace-obliterating obsession with the thin ideal, which, along with dietary perfectionism, is clearly a risk factor for eating pathologies.[8]

Instead of focusing on *weight loss*, I prefer aspiring to realize your *naturally healthy* body. Is it possible that you have been at war with a few "excess" pounds in error? What if you are already at your naturally healthy weight—and I don't mean your fantasy weight, as I demonstrated with my diet counselor? How many more years are you going to continue to tear your hair out over this one? Do you still want to be at war with these same few pounds, fighting hunger, obsessing over it, when you're ninety? Our bodies can regularly fluctuate five to ten pounds anyway, as we all seem to have our own body-defended weight range. Yes, we can impact this positively and sometimes dramatically with our food choices and activity levels—within a certain range. Yet the harder we fight it with suppressed or ignored hunger and deprivation, the more we tend to rebound to a higher defended weight.[9] Maybe you've already proven this to yourself. I know I certainly have.

Dieting can serve as a tangible focus amid life issues that are too overwhelming or complicated to tackle or even acknowledge, distracting you from getting to the core issues. Mindfulness practice puts you in the desired position of being willing to be with and navigate things as they are. That may mean considering you are already where your body wants to be. Or, if not, it can provide a completely different avenue to finding your naturally healthy weight. Even if you are currently carrying a lot of excess poundage, as was I many years back, rather than being laser focused on weight loss, your best ally in becoming your healthiest is to cultivate activity in the regions of the brain that foster awareness, equanimity, patience, emotion regulation, and presence of mind.

It's time we stopped worshipping at the altar of the weight-loss gods, buying into the harm-inducing cultural promotion of body discontent, and indenturing our minds and selling our souls to be thin. There's a better way to find your naturally healthy body and weight. The mindful approach does not force control of food or attempt to *think* your way into changing your eating habits and body. Instead, you transform your relationship to them. Ironically, it wasn't until I let go of the weight loss obsession and, through mindfulness practice, started disarming the reactivity to what life serves up daily that the weight and the painful preoccupation with a "weight problem" itself finally started to fall away.

Disordered Eating and Mindfulness: What the Research Says

In 1999, a study on disordered eating demonstrated that a mindfulness-based intervention can have marked, immediate, and continued impact on episodes of binge eating, as well as associated characteristics such as a perfectionist attitude toward eating, elevated anxiety, distorted and reactive thinking patterns, and a disconnect from hunger and fullness signals. The study showed that the degree to which subjects engaged in mindfulness practice strongly predicted overall improvement. Over the six weeks of the mindfulness program, the number of binge episodes by participants dropped dramatically. Binge size significantly decreased.

Perceived levels of eating control, sense of mindfulness, and awareness of hunger and fullness cues jumped. Anxiety and depression fell.[10]

Results such as these led to more robust studies. A larger study done in 2013 resulted in similar significant changes in behaviors with fewer overeating episodes. It also resulted in weight loss for many participants, though weight loss was not at any time during the study a point of focus. Participants instead focused on regular formal mindfulness meditations, mini mindfulness meditations (such as STOP) throughout the day, and mindful eating.

The more time subjects spent in mindfulness meditation, the greater the benefits. These included getting better at recognizing and paying attention to both hunger and fullness signals, being satisfied with more appropriate amounts of food, a greater sense of control, practicing alternative ways for relieving stress, improved self-esteem, and reduced negative self-judgments.[11] Life-changing shifts such as these are natural outcomes of mindfulness. It starts with the way mindfulness practice increases your ability to not follow through on the impulsive thoughts and urges that run rampant in the chattering, wandering mind.

Does this give us hope for a new way of dealing with cravings, food "addictions," and other unsettling eating urges? You bet. More later in Cravings (page 200) and Addictions (page 213).

⚘ Mindful Moment: Lingering Urges

If you have a long and colorful diet history as I have—one system after another of authoritarian diet systems, behavior checklists, and eating rules that you latched onto only to break—there will be lingering urges to try the same thing again. These urges can be very compelling. After all, as painful as these experiences may have been, they are what you are used to. I can't recall how many times I sat down to read a new diet book over a giant bowl of ice cream. After all, finding a new "system" always brought relief—from the shame, from the feeling of being out of control, from the fear of what the future might bring if I didn't get a grip on my eats. It's an addictive behavior in its own right.

When these thoughts and urges arise, the first point of intervention is to become aware of them. This is very different from identifying with and becoming caught up in them, suppressing them, or trying to negotiate with them. It may be that you are off and running with new dietary regimens for a few minutes before you notice that this is what you are doing. It may show up as a scan of the magazine covers in the checkout line at the market, always eager to lure us into the latest breakthrough magic bullet. At the moment that you become aware of thoughts arising or taking you on a precarious ride, you are experiencing mindfulness. As you become more skilled due to practice, the ability to acknowledge yet not run with these nonproductive thoughts will get stronger. One way I knew that I was getting somewhere is that I lost interest in scanning books or magazines about diets. Boring. What a relief. And the time I got back!

It may be, especially in the early stages, that you will simply go wherever these thoughts want to take you. Yet being aware of the fact that this has taken place is huge. Don't discount the value of this. Just keep up with your formal practice, and intervene in destructive thinking habits as you can. You'll get better at it, I promise.

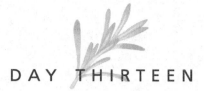

DAY THIRTEEN

becoming vegan

As we shine the light of awareness onto this most ordinary and necessary aspect of our lives—[food]—we shine light onto unperceived chains of bondage attached to our bodies, minds, and hearts, onto the bars of cages we never could quite see, and onto a sparkling path that leads to transformation and the possibility of true love, freedom, and joy in our lives.

—WILL TUTTLE, *The World Peace Diet*

MEDITATION PRACTICE: *13 minutes*

DAY THIRTEEN, *Meditation on Breath and Bodily Sensations*

If you can eat in a way that is endlessly delicious; is beautifully colorful to behold; is most protective of Earth's precious natural resources; builds a resilient, healthy body; and doesn't cause harm to other beings, why wouldn't you choose that? Staying mindful of your reasons for becoming vegan edifies your journey—and meaningful leads to sustainable. Today, we are going to circle back to that moment of awakening, when your heart first opened to the idea of becoming vegan.

Culinary Cofactors

Living vegan builds personal happiness by demonstrating mindfulness in more ways than one:

- **Mindfulness of compassion and ethical sensibility.** You are eating in alignment with your highest ethical ideals. The observation that all sentient beings—people and animals—seek well-being and happiness, rather than suffering and misery, has been made by philosophers and religious thinkers throughout the ages, from Aristotle to Saint Augustine.[1] We have a choice. If we overlook our moral sensitivities and suppress feelings of compassion, inevitably we suffer for it. By eliminating animal products, you are washing your hands of causing harm to animals unnecessarily. You have made the decision not to participate in the needless suffering and demise of billions of creatures—cows, pigs, chickens, turkeys—that takes place every day to satisfy a human desire for meat and dairy. You've embraced the ethic of compassion and opened yourself to experiencing the peace and freedom that come with that.

- **Mindfulness of environmental ethics.** Climate change. Diminished air quality. Habitat destruction. Ocean dead zones. Fisheries depletion. Species extinction. Deforestation. World hunger. Food contamination. There is one issue at the heart of all these problems, too often overlooked by private citizens and policy makers alike—the human-centered, incessant demand for and reliance on animal products.[2] A global shift toward a vegan diet is vital to the world hunger problem and the most serious impacts of climate change.[3]

  Environmental ethics is the defining issue of our times. Inclusive of compassion and personal health, it connects all the dots. In a way, the environmental issue surrounding food choice is of utmost importance. Without a life-supporting planet, there will be no place for either us or the animals to live. As vegan you are also bypassing the dietary "middle man"—meat and other animal products—by eating lower on the food chain. Not only does this mean you circumvent the sidecar of contaminants that bioaccumulate in animal tissues, it is also the single biggest thing you can do to offset pressing environmental and related global issues.[4]

- **Mindfulness of your health.** Eating a plant-foods diet is the biggest player in the prevention and treatment of a long list of diseases: coronary artery disease, diabetes, hypertension, obesity, and certain forms of cancer.[5] In other words, you don't eat one diet for preventing heart disease, another for obesity, and yet another for diabetes. Eating a healthy vegan diet is positively protective of your health across the board.[6] It's also the best way to find your naturally healthy weight.

Vegan, Plant-Based, Or...

To clarify the terminology, *plant-based* literally means the majority— if not all—of the energy from the food you eat comes from plants. Technically, there could possibly be smidgens of animal products in the diet—the errant chunk of cheese, the occasional slice of turkey—and you'd still be eating plant-based. Some people who describe their diet as plant-based include small portions of animal products purposely, while others eschew all animal products.

The term *vegan* draws a different picture; it aspires to exclude animal products in other forms, not just diet. This could still, however, mean an unhealthy diet, full of highly processed foods. My preferred term is *healthy vegan* because it is just what it says. *Healthy*—from eating plant-exclusive, whole, primarily minimally processed food. *Vegan* considers also the health of the planet and the other sentient beings we share it with—and the holistic health that comes with choosing not to participate in the duplicity of professing a love of animals while seeing them as a commodity or objects of consumption.

Some people prefer the term *plant-based*, saying it describes more what is included rather than excluded. Yet in the bigger picture, *healthy vegan* underscores what's included. For along with the plants on your plate come care, compassion, ethical alignment, joy, freedom, responsibility, vision, clear conscience, integrity, cognitive resonance, and peace.

Vegan Is Visionary

Eating a healthy vegan diet, you are ahead of the curve. So why didn't your doctor tell you? If eating well can help prevent chronic conditions, one has to wonder, why aren't more physicians prescribing broccoli and Brazil nuts? As important a role modern medicine can play in public health, shouldn't we be partnering our pharmacies with farmacies? Take two red peppers and call me in the morning? We've known for years that doctors receive precious little nutrition education in medical school. Isn't it about time for that deficit to shift?

Fortunately, that nutrition training gap may be narrowing. Due to the dramatic expansion of the science surrounding the connections between nutrition, health, and disease over the last several decades—which consistently points to the benefits to our bodies of eating more fruits, vegetables, whole grains, legumes, and nuts and less of everything else—disease prevention and health promotion are becoming prioritized by policy makers and payers.[7] That includes medical school curricula reform to increase nutrition education—and calls to action for doctors to learn how to translate diet and lifestyle knowledge to you and me.[8] Finally! Once you know that you don't have to cause harm to yourself, or the animals, or pillage the environment in order to enjoy delicious food, becoming vegan is an easy choice.

⚘ Mindful Moment: Intention Investigation

What has inspired you to become vegan? It's likely that one of the reasons described here has played a part in your decision to change your life in this most fundamental way. Perhaps your original reason for going vegan has spilled over into one or more of the other areas, multiplying your motivation.

Think back to that moment in time when you were first awakened to the idea of becoming vegan. What was the circumstance? Who were you with? Was it a film, a conversation overheard, a book? Something on social media? A leaflet? Conviction that simply emerged from within as you became awake to what it meant to have a piece of animal on your plate? Each of us has a story to tell. What is yours?

Now, dig a little deeper. What is the intention, core value, or ethic that is expressed in your choices? For example, when I became vegetarian more than forty-five years ago, my reasons were nonviolence and moral ethics, concern for the environment, and health. These reasons have become even more compelling over time.

Establishing intention can clarify the choices you make every day. It creates a mindful link with why you do what you do, edifying your practices. It gives you a lens to detect inconsistencies that you may be sensing in your own life yet haven't seen clearly. It helps bring what you do more in alignment with what is important to you. This can be valuable for authentic conversations with others who are interested in why you make the choices that you do. It doesn't make you perfect at it. Yet your mindfulness practice will fundamentally improve the connection and reinforce your skills at following through. In the words of my friend Ari Nessel, founder of The Pollination Project:

> When a person adopts a vegan lifestyle for moral reasons, they are touching into the quality of compassion and the wish for sufferings of others to diminish. For me, cultivating this quality is half the way to living a fulfilling and joyful life. The other half comes from developing wisdom, the ability to renounce that which causes us, and eventually others, pain. I have found no other practice more effective in cultivating wisdom than mindfulness (or meditation in its more formal practice). Mindfulness is the key to seeing my own patterns and identifying what thoughts, words, and deeds serve others and myself. It creates the space between stimulus and response that allows me to choose how I show up in the world, rather than just have knee-jerk reactions to life.[9]

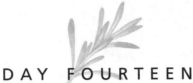

the mindful vegan plate

Our choices are more about compassion than personal purity.
—BRENDA DAVIS, RD

MEDITATION PRACTICE: *14 minutes*

DAY FOURTEEN, *Meditation on Breath and Bodily Sensations*

Being mindful also includes mindfulness of how what you eat affects your health—upon which eating a plant-based diet has a proven positive effect. Yet if the terms *healthy vegan* or *plant-based* conjure up visions of grass with a side of twigs and bark, it's time to set the story straight. In today's lesson, you will discover a simple primer for what foods are in the giant basket labeled "healthy vegan."

Mindfulness of Health

Yes, it's beneficial to eat lots of leafy green vegetables. Yet they aren't enough on their own to satisfy your appetite or give you the energy you need. The mindful vegan plate is not only rich in color and fiber, it's also abundant in flavor, pleasure, eye appeal, appetite satisfaction, and the original comfort foods. Along with the bright rainbow of colors in salads and stir-fries, why not enjoy:

- mashed potatoes, yams, corn, muffins, and mounds of steamy whole grains
- bowls of savory lentil soup with sourdough bread
- mushroom meatballs on a pile of pasta or swimming in a savory marinara or mushroom sauce
- black bean enchiladas with salsa and guacamole
- teriyaki tofu on a bed of black rice
- platters of your favorite fruits—apples, mangoes, melons, berries—and handfuls of your favorite nuts and seeds

Make sure there are plenty of satisfying legumes, starches, and fruits on your plate along with the colorful vegetables and salads and nuts or seeds. Now you're talking healthy, happy human.

The Core Players on the Mindful Plate

These foods form the foundation of optimal nutrition. Center your meals on primarily whole plant foods, minimally processed. That means the original parts of the plant are present—even if they are altered slightly by being chopped, cracked, ground, cooked, or blended. This opens up an endless variety of what's for dinner.

Rather than give you meal plans and serving sizes, tell you how much raw versus cooked food to eat, or sideline the conversation in any other fashion, the healthy vegan plate is presented here to keep it simple and clear about what foods to focus on for health. Keep these at the center of your choices.

Reasonable Regulars and Occasional Others

What about birthday cake, pumpkin pie, and vegan ice cream? Do your favorite sourdough bread, salad dressing, nondairy cheese, and champagne fit in? What about that soy cappuccino? I enjoy these, too. Rather

The Mindful Vegan Plate
These foods and more—
and everything made from them!

Beans and Legumes: adzuki beans, black beans, black-eyed peas, cannellini beans, chickpeas, kidney beans, lentils, lima beans, peanuts, pinto beans, soybeans/edamame, split peas, tempeh, tofu, white beans

Whole Grains: amaranth, barley, buckwheat, corn, kamut, millet, oats, polenta, quinoa, rye, rice, spelt, wheat; cracked grains such as bulgur; whole-grain breads, whole-wheat couscous, whole-grain flours, whole-grain pasta

Vegetables: acorn squash, artichokes, arugula, asparagus, basil, beets, bok choy, broccoli, Brussels sprouts, butternut squash, cabbage, carrots, cauliflower, celery, collard greens, corn, cucumber, eggplant, green beans, green onion, kale, lettuce, mushrooms, mustard greens, okra, olives, parsley, peas, peppers, potatoes, rhubarb, romaine, spinach, sweet potatoes, Swiss chard, zucchini

Fruits: apples, avocados, bananas, berries, cherries, grapes, grapefruits, kiwis, lemons, mandarins, mangoes, melons, oranges, papayas, peaches, pears, pomegranates

Nuts and Seeds: almonds, Brazil nuts, cashews, coconuts, flaxseeds, hazelnuts, hemp seeds, nut and seed butters, peanuts (officially a legume), pecans, pine nuts, pistachios, sesame seeds, sunflower seeds, walnuts

than imply that these treats are forbidden and that you should never indulge, or lead you to believe I never do, I'll keep it real. It's important to keep this reasonable, easy, and fun.

Depending on where you are on your vegan journey and the occasion that has presented itself, there's plenty of room for what I call "reasonable regulars" and "occasional others." Of course, should you have specific health concerns, be mindful of them. If there are certain foods, meal timing protocols, or other considerations that you have found beneficial to your health, your mindfulness practice can make it possible for you to follow through on maintaining them with greater ease.

Some people are strictly legalistic when it comes to processed versus unprocessed. This can perpetuate a tension-around-eating problem that can backfire, triggering dietary disinhibition. In plain English, that means the "what the hell" factor. This compulsive letting go of all controls is extremely disheartening. In knee-jerk fashion, it can cause you to attempt drawing an even firmer line over which you swear not to cross. The result can be a heightened struggle because you are essentially trying to solve the problem *at the level at which it was created*—reactivity and impulsiveness. Signing off on a food mandate means nothing without the presence of mind to back it up. Mindfulness, while enhancing follow-through, frees you from perfectionism.

Reasonable Regulars

Ketchup on your veggie burger, cooking wine in your stir-fry, teriyaki sauce for your tofu—these may not fit into the "whole foods" description. But that doesn't mean they aren't players on the plate of what you enjoy every day. And let's not forget, enjoying what you eat is important. Another example of reasonable regulars is plant milk, which has often had its fiber filtered out. That doesn't mean you need to yank it off your table. A splash of soy milk on your morning bowl of grains, or coconut milk added to the blender in a green smoothie or to the food processor to make ice cream (see Vegan Cherry Garcia, page 263), is a perfect example of a reasonable regular. This is not the same as chugging down a big glass of almond milk at each meal. Yet it's enough to add delight, delectableness, and ease to your healthy vegan fare. Even if a regular player, it is in reasonable amounts relative to the whole plant foods that form the core of what you eat.

Occasional Others

Can you really enjoy that decadent vegan cake on your birthday, the chocolate mousse pie during the holidays, and the occasional vegan cheese pizza splurge? Won't this send you on a vegan junk food tailspin?

Eating à la mindful vegan means that while you are aware of the health implications of what you eat, you also enjoy freedom from authoritarian food lists that lock you out of eating vegan treats at celebrations, special events, and even the occasional hedonic moment. Yet that's why they are called occasional others. In my dieting days—including several months in Overeaters Anonymous—I followed several diet regimens that had me draw a bright line around certain treats because I thought they fueled my "addiction" to sweets. Ironically, the only way I discovered my naturally healthy weight was through the process of letting go of so many controls around food. When I started mindfulness meditation practice, embraced mindful living and eating, and gave up dieting, portions-by-scale, and undereating—and stopped seeing myself as powerless over food—my world transformed.

Another example of occasional others is nudging the whole-food line as it may present itself at family and social events. For example, recently my husband, Greg, and I were invited to dinner at a friend's home. Though I always tell the host in advance that we're happy with rice, beans, and a big bowl of salad for dinner, once we arrived, we discovered that our hostess had gone to great lengths to prepare an extravagant vegan meal. Much fancier, with richer ingredients than what I use at home, it was more like something I would reserve for a holiday feast. She had not only done her Sherlock Holmes best at the local market to make sure the lasagna noodles she was using had no animal products, she had also driven to the next town to procure some specialty vegan cheese to use. Heavens!

Sticking to the center circle of optimal nutrition in this circumstance is not what was called for. What was important was focusing on how happy we were that she had prepared for us such a lovely vegan meal, and how delicious it was. This puts the focus on where it matters. It is compassionate and kind to the hostess. It makes eating vegan look exactly like what it is—fun, easy, and a happy experience.

Mindful eating opens up a joyous new perspective. It disentangles you from the debilitating, stifling fear of special occasions and treats. As your mindfulness practice continues, your ability to select skillfully, and the freedom to do so, grows. You gain the power of choice—and that means choosing to indulge, choosing not to indulge, and being at ease with it all.

Keep It Simple

Some people get distracted from the simple basics of a healthy vegan diet by engaging in an exhausting overanalysis of nutrients. Such dietary acrobatics—trying to make sure to get just the right amount of this or that nutrient every day—aren't necessary. Worrying about this kind of precision can get in the way of enjoying your meals and hamper your ability to stay the vegan course.

Others become preoccupied with eating only organic or local fare. These may be important players as you advance your journey. Yet if you are obsessing about your broccoli being not only organic but local, fresh, and non-GMO—and can't find it even after driving all over town to track some down—remember the important thing here: eating some broccoli. Aspiring to eat ten or more servings of vegetables and fruits a day? Smart. Being mindful of having plenty of legumes and whole grains or other quality starch- and protein-rich foods on your plate? Simply good sense. Tracking every nutrient and all the minutiae at mealtime? Not so much. It is more important to delight in simple, great-tasting healthy food and to be mindfully present with your plate so that you don't miss a single delicious bite. Keep your favorite fruits and vegetables on hand. Let go of trying to force yourself to eat those you don't like, while at the same time be open to adventure into new veggie territory.

Being present with your meal is also the pathway to attuning to your natural hunger and fullness signals, which—along with a predominance of minimally processed foods—will guide you to your naturally healthy body and weight. Be mindful of eating a variety of foods primarily from the nutritionally optimal, healthy vegan core over time. Variety helps insure that you get a wide spectrum of nutrients—including the all-important antioxidants, fiber, and all the other phytonutrients that plants deliver.

Numbers Game?

Perhaps you feel compelled to control your food in other ways, such as precise proportions or counting calories. While having awareness of the energy density of various foods is wise, obsessing with the calorie count on your plate pulls your attention away from mindfulness of fullness and getting true satisfaction from your meal. If this sounds like you, can you honestly say that calorie counting has been successful for you in sustaining your naturally healthy weight? More importantly, has it helped you build a happy relationship with food and your body?

Sarah, a client of mine, comes to mind. Struggling with her food and weight, Sarah came to me for help. During our first conversation, almost the first thing she said was, "Don't make me give up my calorie counting! It's the only way I have control!" Sarah proceeded to describe to me how she would eat "very carefully" for a few days. She would count her calories religiously, writing every calorie count down. But after about five days, she would "lose control" and wildly overeat. On these days, Sarah told me, she abandoned calorie counting.

I asked Sarah how long this pattern had been playing itself out.

"For years!" she said. Was calorie counting giving Sarah control? Or was it giving her the illusion of control, while in actuality creating more distance between Sarah, a peaceful relationship with eating, a connection with her hunger and fullness signals, and her naturally healthy weight?

I couldn't fault Sarah, as at one time I, too, was obsessed with calorie counting. I got so good at it that I could do it in my sleep. But after a while, it took on a life of its own. Every plate of food was a numbers project, giving me the illusion of control and sucking all the joy out of the meal. It blocked any possibility of eating according to natural signals of hunger and fullness by keeping me in my head and out of my body's mealtime experience. It didn't solve my weight problem more than temporarily.

✿ Mindful Moment: Mealtime Math

While mindful living includes being aware of the overall nutritional balance and wholesomeness of your meals, turning each repast into a math project can destroy a good meal. Preoccupation with the details, such as obsessing over nutrient balance or counting one thing or another, creates unnecessary anxiety. It perpetuates a punitive perspective of your plate, hampers the connection with your fullness signals, and disconnects you from taking real pleasure in your food. If you have a history of micromanaging your diet, a carryover from food plans you've followed in days gone by, the urge to gain control through some kind of counting system may surprise you with its urgency. This is simply because what you have reinforced through practice has become the default habit of the mind. Your brain has hardwired mealtime with math time.

Mindfulness practice gives you the keys to get out of the counting cage. When these thoughts—the urge to count or otherwise force control—arise, mentally note them. Then, utilize the skills you have been practicing in formal mindfulness practice to allow them to pass right by on the thought train. Notice the sensations in your body that signal to you your interest in the topic. If you are deeply used to this kind of micromanagement, you may notice a restlessness or fear in your body characterized by tension, accompanied by an overwhelming urge to comply by counting. Let these bodily sensations be a momentary point of investigation for you, further acknowledging the rising of thoughts without reinforcing them. Don't suppress the thoughts or sensations, or try to push them away. Simply observe curiously, with a willingness to be with whatever has presented itself. You will probably notice the thoughts will give way to something else, and the tension in your body will be released. They may come back, repeatedly, until a new, stronger pattern has been developed.

If abandoning controls such as counting calories is too much for you to pass on right away, you can approach letting these habits go via making microchanges while you develop a greater degree of mastery over where you invest your thought energy. Here's how I disentangled myself from an obsession with calorie counting. At first, complete abandonment of it brought up too much fear. So, I told myself that I could go ahead and count calories, but not until evening when I was done eating for the day. This way I acknowledged the mental pull to engage in the count yet gently turned over the controls of how much to eat to my body, via mindful eating. After a while, I started skipping the end-of-the-day count more and more often as I let go of it in favor of my higher aspiration of eating mindfully according to my body's fuel signals. This compassionate approach served me well.

At the same time, if counting or measuring is doctor ordered, far be it from me to suggest otherwise. In that case, to increase enjoyment and relaxation around meal time, take note of your emotions and inner condition when the count ensues. Do you ruminate or obsess about it? What does that feel like? Is any tension around food created during the process? Should you decide to keep up the practice of tracking in this manner, you can utilize mindfulness skills to view your food through this lens with greater relaxation and ease.

More on Vegan Nutrition

If you are looking for deeper assistance with transitioning to healthy vegan eating, *The Plant-Based Journey: A Step-by-Step Guide to Transitioning to a Healthy Lifestyle and Achieving Your Ideal Weight* (BenBella Books, 2015) is a guide written specifically for that purpose. Transition timelines, systems for success, multiple recipe templates, getting the family on board, and the Easy Meal Planner—they're all there.

Perhaps you are interested in diving deeper into the study of vegan nutrition. Maybe you have particular nutritional needs, food sensitivities, or simply a desire to find out more about the science of a healthy vegan diet. My go-to guide, and the gold standard for vegan nutrition, is *Becoming Vegan* (Book Publishing Co., 2014) by Brenda Davis, RD, and Vesanto Melina, RD. Vegan quick starter guides can be found at vegan.com/nutrition/, brendadavisrd.com/the-vegan-plate/, as well as many others in Resources at themindfulveganbook.com.

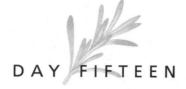

DAY FIFTEEN

meditation on emotions

Healing and freedom come from non-proliferation of our thoughts. Non-proliferation means we have the wisdom in our lives to pause and re-arrive in the present moment.
In that manner we can tap the wisdom and the kindness that is intrinsic to our nature. We then can respond with intelligence instead of a kind of fear-based reaction.

—TARA BRACH

 MEDITATION PRACTICE: *15 minutes*

🔊 *Day Fifteen, Meditation on Emotions*

The next adventure for mindfulness practice steps into the realm of emotions. This builds directly upon the experiences and tools of observation that you are utilizing with the breath and bodily sensation meditations. Emotions register in your physical body, too—after all, we call them "feelings." These practices—the meditation on the breath, bodily sensations, and emotions—together improve your mindfulness of the present moment.

With mindfulness of emotions, you add an important element to your practice. For most of us, our day is a string of reactions to a series of emotions that can accompany thoughts or arise on their own. Mindfulness improves your discernment of emotional states. It is here, in mindfulness of emotion, that you further develop the tools that lead to the mechanics of shifting from reactivity to response.

Mindfully accepting an emotion doesn't mean that you wallow in it or act on it irresponsibly. Quite the opposite. Rather than being driven by unexamined habit, the more directly you connect with your feelings, the more effectively proactive you can become. You increase your ability to make better, more skillful choices. Until you can acknowledge a thought or emotion as part of your human repertoire—observe it to see that it won't last forever, that it isn't all that you are—you can't create a healthy relationship to it.

Mindfulness and Embodiment of Emotions

Every experience we have is registered emotionally, accompanied by a physical correlate in your body. For this reason, as embodiment of your emotional experiences, your body can teach you more than you realize. Physical sensations are the currency of our unconscious processing of emotion. Mindfulness gives you tools to listen to, navigate, and respond to emotions skillfully.

To give you an example of how emotions are reflected in your body, try this simple exercise. Recall a recent moment when you felt really angry. Okay, do you have it? Recalling the situation may re-create the same anger—perhaps to a lesser or even greater degree—than when it occurred. For the sake of this exercise, it doesn't matter. Now, take your attention from your (what I am sure was justified) angry thoughts and shift your focus to your body. How do you *know* you were angry? Where does anger show up, physically? Do you feel tightness in your chest, a knot in your stomach, tension in your face, or constriction at the throat? Do you notice tension in other areas of your body?

Try the same exercise with feelings of happiness. Think back to a recent moment when you felt really happy. Maybe you were on a quiet walk and felt joyfully connected with nature. Maybe a loved one did or said something especially thoughtful. Maybe your dog ran up and gave you a big sloppy kiss. You felt happy. How did you *know* you were happy? Was there an opening in your heart, a flutter in your stomach, brightness in your countenance? These sensations are the embodiment of emotions—the avenue through which you work with them during both formal practice and informal practice.

Wheel of Emotions

Most of our feelings arise from a combination of life encounters and genetic factors. Robert Plutchik's wheel of emotions is one representation of the range and variations-on-a-theme that are part of our emotional experience.

Awareness of this range of emotions can help us gain clarity on our experience of "feelings." As we start to work with them in mindfulness practice, we discover an interesting truth—emotions and feelings rarely last more than several seconds, if minutes, before being replaced

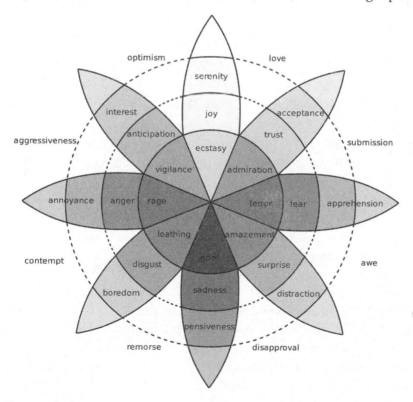

by another. More important than identifying them each time one surfaces is the fact that you can detect the differences between them, recognize their qualities, and note their changing. That means there is some inner space around each of them—space where mindfulness of them can be cultivated. This is precisely where you can move from emotional reactivity to skillful response. With mindfulness meditation practice, you are cultivating the capacity to experience thoughts, feelings, and other phenomena without adding a layer of judgment or elaboration. This makes it possible to recognize the field of awareness surrounding each such event, opening up territory between stimulus and automatic reactions.[1]

Maybe you have stellar skills for managing emotions. But most of us never got an education about how to work with them in a way that is helpful. In my own experience, I recall the distinct feeling that though happiness was fine, anger was an emotion largely unacceptable to express. Whether this was true or not, in my early years I cultivated many ways to bury or deny angry feelings. This resulted in lots of inner confusion, stress, sadness, blindsiding outbursts, and baffling eating behaviors.

Mindfulness and Emotional Self-Regulation

Though we often try to figure out why we may be thinking or feeling a certain way—and these investigations can be helpful processes as an adjunct to mindfulness—meditation practice is the time for working with these feelings in a direct way rather than with discursive analysis. With mindfulness practice, you usher in a new era of acceptance of your emotions by acknowledging, recognizing, and allowing yourself to experience their presence. *This is not the same as getting caught up in them*, where they can lead you to act them out in ways that are befuddling to yourself or harmful to others. Instead of either repressing them or getting carried away by them, with mindfulness you learn to see emotions as you do thoughts and physical sensations—as phenomena. They are important though temporary experiences, with tremendous power to inform you yet also negatively affect your physical and mental states. They can increase anxiety, sadness, and depression—feelings that are, according to clinical research, reduced among those that practice mindfulness meditation.[2]

Mindful emotion regulation represents the capacity to remain aware. Again, this does not mean suppression of the emotional experience or attempts to alter emotions in any way. With mindfulness meditation you experience a retraining of your awareness coupled with nonreactivity. This allows you to more consciously choose responses to emotions, disassembling the automatic process of reactivity that can give rise to disturbing emotions in the first place. In the bigger picture, through this process you increasingly connect with the awareness that underlies all mental phenomena. As this occurs, a number of positive emotions and traits emerge—your inherent qualities of compassion, equanimity, patience, kindness. You reinforce your facility for mindfulness.[3] The outcome? An increased capacity for taking more appropriate action on righting wrongs, speaking up with clarity and compassion, and acknowledging reactivity and your own blind spots. This translates to living with greater ease and communicating more confidently.

Emotional reactivity is in many ways an evolutionary bonus. Being easily alerted to danger is an important survival mechanism, as we differentiate the snakes from the sticks. Yet we all know that the nature of emotional reactivity can be problematic in certain situations if allowed to operate unconsciously and unregulated. Excessive rumination, out-of-control worry—these are examples with which we can all easily relate. Some degree of management of these otherwise reflexive processes can be of enormous benefit, bringing relief to the misery caused by runaway emotional reaction.

Meditation on Emotions

Begin the Meditation on Emotions in the same way as every mindfulness practice: position, anchor, intention, and remindfulness. Continue with mindfulness of breath for a few minutes to assist concentration.

Now, expand your awareness to the sensations of the body, just as you have been practicing in meditation of bodily sensations. You can do a quick body survey if you like, or simply become globally aware of any sensations that are showing up in your body right now. Maybe you feel a tingling in your hands or feet. It is important not to specifically look for anything or try to create something. Just increase your attentive connection with what is showing up right now.

Next, take a few moments to notice your emotional state. How are you feeling? What's your mood? There is always some emotional state or mood present, even if you don't recognize it. Maybe there is a feeling of happiness, or sadness, or restlessness. How do you know that you are feeling happy, or sad, or any other emotion? What sensations do you notice in your body right now that are giving you information about your emotions—the direct experience of it? How are you relating to the emotion you are experiencing?

Though they subtly reverberate throughout your system, emotions usually show up most prominently as sensations in the core of the body. We don't feel sadness in our knees, for example. We usually feel emotions in the throat, the chest, the belly—the center of your emotional body. To help connect with your current state of emotions, you can do a body survey that focuses on these areas. After all, these are bodily sensations, too—they are just showing up on another level. Bring your attention to the throat and upper chest to shine a light on what emotions you may be experiencing. Is there a constriction or lump in the throat? From there, you can investigate the chest for any sensations connected with emotions. Perhaps a tightness, or an expansive feeling, or heaviness. Investigate the stomach area. Any tension, knots, butterflies? These are all emotions that are showing up as physical sensations. Note also if you have any judgments, thoughts, ideas, or reactions to your mood state or emotion.

Let your attention rest on whichever of these emotional indicators is the strongest. Just as with the breath and the bodily sensations, observe these sensations with bare attention. Do the sensations grow, shrink, change? Is there a temperature to them? Are they moving around, or vibrating? Without looking for a specific sensation, just see what is there. Can you identify the emotion that the sensations are conveying? If so, you can briefly use mental noting, such as "sadness," or "happiness," or "anxiety." This is not the time to get wrapped up in a debate about which emotion you are experiencing; noting can simply assist awareness. Quickly, return your attention to the sensations themselves. Continue to be present with how the feeling of emotions is showing up, if and how it changes, if it gets stronger, weaker, disappears, or changes to something altogether different—all of which are possible.

You may find that bringing your attention to the sensations of emotion in this fashion makes you want to figure them out, push them away, or get involved in a story around what may have caused them. This is perhaps the most challenging aspect of meditation on emotions—the pull to get caught up in the drama around them. Note these urges just as you have been noting thoughts in your mindfulness of breath and bodily sensations meditations. Acknowledge them, and gently—with kindness, patience, and equanimity—return your attention to the sensations of the emotion.

If you start to feel lost or disoriented, or observing your emotions starts to feel overwhelming, you can gently return to your old friend, the breath, as anchor. And if your mind wanders—which it will—you can return your attention to the breath anchor to recover attentive aware-ness. You can return to meditation on the sensations of emotions when and if you are ready. If you prefer, you can stay with the breath as anchor through the rest of today's sitting. As you continue your meditation, being relaxed, at ease, and keeping a sense of kindness toward yourself and these sensations is central. In the days ahead, meditation on emo-tions will be incorporated into the practices of meditation on the breath and bodily sensations. Today, we're just dipping our toes in the pool to learn more about how sensations connected with emotions can occur throughout the body—some pleasant, some unpleasant—continually arising and passing away in a continuous process of change.

Finally, return your attention once again to the feeling of the breath. Bring loving kindness to yourself for whatever you are feeling right now. Holding yourself in this kindness, gently open your eyes. Set an inten-tion to bring some of this quality of kindness and mindfulness forward with you into your day.

Mindful Moment: Minding Your Emotions

Our default reaction to emotions tends to have love-hate qualities. We lean toward wanting to keep the positive feelings and get rid of the negative ones. We get caught up in evaluations of our emotions, automatically triggering negative self-judgment and gloomy moods. Mindfulness redirects your attention to sensations, away from evaluation. By cultivating bare attention—simply remaining attentive to what is showing up, without expectation—to present moment sensation, mindfulness presents you with a task that does not require deployment of your evaluating faculties.

Instead of suppressing feelings, pushing them away, or getting caught up in them, mindfulness builds emotional self-regulation by establishing new pathways in the brain that offer an alternative.[4] By explicitly practicing a willingness to be fully present, you begin to recognize whatever is presenting itself, without participating in making judgment calls on your sensory experiences. This practice not only increases emotional awareness, it also disrupts activity in certain parts of the brain that lead to distress. It invites self-compassion, acceptance, and the ability to navigate and respond more skillfully to emotions. It inspires equanimity. You can walk right through the middle of mental and emotional states and emerge with insights and the ability to make more skillful choices.

Don't be surprised if at some point an insight to the source of these emotions pops up. This is different from investigating them intellectually, and it can come unbidden as an organic outcome of your investigation. You may suddenly be flooded with a memory, or have some flash of understanding about it. These are very helpful moments of wisdom that only come about because you bypassed intellectualizing about the moment to go to direct experience. It is one of the reasons this kind of meditation is also called insight meditation.

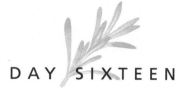

RAIN

*Equanimity is the balanced, non-reactive mind and heart,
grounded in wisdom, and filled with a spaciousness that leads
to an appropriate response.*

—HEATHER SUNDBERG, Insight Meditation Teacher

MEDITATION PRACTICE: *16 minutes*

DAY SIXTEEN, *RAIN; Meditation on Breath and Bodily Sensations*

The mindful approach to emotions may well be unlike anything you have ever experienced before. I know it has been for me. It has also proven to be the single biggest agency for personal change for me because of the tools it delivers for navigating emotions, reactivity in everything from food to conversations, and life's daily ups and downs. It has established a fundamental equanimity that gets rattled far less than it used to.

When in our schooling did we ever learn how to steer our way through emotions? No wonder we struggle with confused states and baffling habits, without a clue as to how to implement a better way—or even know that one exists.

Emotions can seem so compelling and inseparable from our experience, it can be hard to imagine finding any space around them, let

133

alone figure out how to navigate them. We all differ in our ability to regulate emotion. Some of us simply have stronger emotional self-regulation skills, whether from genetics or from learning it by being around someone as we were growing up who skillfully managed emotion.

Today, you'll learn RAIN, an acronym for the four steps of a process that gives you a place to turn to in a painful, volatile, or otherwise unsettling moment. RAIN directs your attention in a clear, systematic way that plies through confusion and stress. As you call on RAIN with more regularity, this mindful practice brings a new calm and quality of openness to your daily life.

RAIN

RAIN—recognition, acknowledgement and acceptance, investigation, and nonidentification—is a superpractical, sequential, in-the-trenches process for working with emotions. It establishes a clear and profound connection between your formal mindfulness practice and the rest of your day outside of formal practice. Here is how to use the RAIN method to navigate emotionally challenging moments.

Recognition

The moment of recognition is the very second you notice that you are in the grip of a strong emotion or are caught in reactivity. It needn't be something big—misplaced keys, something said then quickly regretted, unwashed dishes, one cookie too many—all can be enough to trigger reactivity. Recognition is the first step to being mindful in the midst of your emotions. You may even be well into the experience of an emotion before you become mindful of its presence. It may already have manifested as bodily tension, changes in your breathing pattern or heart rate, your posture and body language—or a sudden outburst. When you recognize you are caught up in reactivity, pause and take a breath or two to help you disengage from the momentum of the moment. As you progress with mindfulness practice, the moment of recognition will come much earlier in the process of the emotional experience—perhaps before you are aware of it in thought.

Acknowledgment and Acceptance

This step of the RAIN process is an extension of the basic tenet of mindfulness, which brings to your experience a kind and accepting attitude. We often sit in judgment of our emotions, reactions, and thoughts. We easily get caught up in them or, in the case of difficult emotions, push them away. After all, who wants to experience the feelings around a bad breakup, the pinch of regret, or the sudden misfortune of someone close to us? Yet when we engage in an inner struggle in this way, we unknowingly create more suffering and tension.

Acknowledging what you are experiencing emotionally doesn't mean that you like it or that you are saying it's a good or bad thing. Not at all. But you can become mindful of these moments and acknowledge that they are passing through you as part of your experience. By allowing this, you're able to bring an inner "yes, this is what is happening" to your present moment. You may notice almost immediately a sense of softening and ease around the emotion as you let go of the resistance in favor of willing to be present.

Investigation

Once you have recognized and accepted the presence of an emotion, you investigate what the emotion feels like in your body. This is where you employ curiosity. How does the feeling manifest itself? How do you know you are angry, sad, anxious, excited, happy? This is the most powerful moment in the RAIN process, yet it necessitates going through the first two steps to get to this point. It's also the trickiest because it is very tempting to get lost in the story that drummed up the emotion in the first place.

For example, let's say a coworker blamed you for something of which you are completely innocent, inspiring indignation—and rightfully so! You may find that you keep returning to the event that instigated the emotion. "How dare he say that!" and "Who does she think she is?" and "How could he do that after all I've done to . . ." It goes on and on. And whether true or not, the point is this tendency of the mind is derailing the investigative process. It doesn't mean that you cave, buckle to abuse, or become a doormat at work. This isn't outer conflict management; it's inner conflict management, so that you can restore some sense of equanimity in the full face of the situation. This will far better position you for taking more skillful action in outer management.

The other tricky element of the investigative stage is the temptation to try to figure out why you are feeling a certain way, or to "think about" the emotion, what in your past may have caused you to hook into it, and so on. These may be helpful processes, yet now is not the time. Save these inquiries for another time, outside of the RAIN process. You can explore them later in thought, a conversation with a friend, reflective writing, or even therapy. Keep your attention on the physical sensations you are experiencing.

Not everyone can sense the feeling of emotion in their body right away. For example, during a recent instruction on mindfulness that I was giving, the group was in the midst of an activity we did in yesterday's lesson—recalling an experience of anger and noticing the sensations in the body. There were about two hundred people in the room, and everyone was on board with "feeling" their anger except for one gentleman. He insisted he could not feel anything in his body that was reflecting his anger. Yet he was, obvious to everyone else in the room, quite keyed up. There was visible tension on his face and throughout his body, his shoulders hunching as he recalled his anger at the desk clerk at the hotel earlier that day.

In trying to help him navigate the physical experience around the anger, I repeated, "How did you *know* you were angry?"

His response was, "Because I yelled at the clerk!" But he could not sense the bodily reflection of anger that was so visible to the rest of us.

If you are having trouble connecting with bodily sensations, first and foremost, understand that you are doing nothing wrong. Everyone is on their own journey into connecting with these phenomena, and as you continue with your practice, this link with bodily sensation will grow. You can try to notice any general sense the emotion is giving you. For example, ask yourself the question—does it feel like fear? Does it feel like sadness? Stay attentive yet compassionate, open to anything that shows up. The most important thing here is pausing, deepening your attention, and regarding yourself with kindness and patience as much as possible.

The point of being mindful with emotions is not to seek a certain experience, to try to make the emotions go away, or to look for deep insights into your childhood. The idea is to become aware of the emotions to the best of your ability and how they manifest in your body in the present moment. Through this process, you will naturally find yourself at the next step.

Nonidentification

The first three steps of RAIN allow the fourth to come by itself. At this step you grow increasingly aware that you are not your emotions. Rather, you embody the quality of awareness that is present to be aware of every emotion, sense perception, or even thought for that matter. Nonidentification means that your sense of who you are is not irrevocably fused with or defined by your emotions and thoughts. By not taking your emotions so personally, you create some space around them so that you eventually relax the grip of getting all caught up in and carried away by them—which can be the cause of great personal misery. Rather, the emotions are something passing through you. Emotion = energy in motion.

As you disidentify from the contents of consciousness such as thoughts and feelings, you can view your moment-by-moment experiences with greater objectivity. This is a fundamental shift in perspective. Rather than being caught up in the drama of a personal narrative, you are able to stand back and simply bear witness. For example, if anxiety arises, and you strongly identify with it, there will be a greater tendency to react to the anxiety with old habits and try to regulate it with some unskillful behavior, such as stress eating, drinking, zoning out online, or going on a shopping spree. Nonidentification lets you step back from the anxiety and see it clearly as simply an emotional state that is arising and that will eventually pass away. This knowledge of the impermanence of mental and emotional phenomena allows a higher level of tolerance for unpleasant internal states.[1]

Nonidentification can be a difficult concept to understand intellectually yet, once experienced, makes perfect sense. We can have flashes of it at first. Chances are you may have had glimpses of it already, even before undertaking mindfulness practice, when you experienced a difficult emotion and yet you knew, deep inside, that somehow you'd be okay. In that moment, you were experiencing disidentification. Don't worry, this doesn't turn you into a zombie or an automaton. Far from it. It is the automaticity that we are moving away from in this process, into a genuine experience of the present. You are moving through it more skillfully so that your emotions don't bounce back to bite you later because you ran from them, suppressed them, impulsively acted them out, or obsessed over what caused them. Such are our usual default mechanisms that can cause so much difficulty.

Often the emotion we are experiencing isn't so much the problem as is the meaning we give to it. For example, it's the difference between thinking "I am feeling so nervous" and "I'm a nervous wreck!" RAIN helps us loosen our grip on the emotion, and its grip on us.

As you become more practiced, these steps can take place with lightning speed. You'll start the investigative process by instinct because the recognition and acknowledgment become almost automatic.

❀ Mindful Moment: Weather Patterns

Emotions are like weather patterns. Sometimes the weather is cloudy, sometimes stormy, and at other times sunny. Sometimes they hit us unexpectedly like a rain squall. At other times we can see the storm clouds gather. Sometimes we know why we are feeling a certain way. And sometimes there is no rhyme or reason why we are experiencing a certain emotion, or have any idea of where it has come from. Maybe an emotion out of nowhere is simply the process of something from your past unfolding. It may have been triggered by something you saw, heard, even tasted. I remember once bursting into tears during a massage, apparently because it unearthed a buried emotion; though the experienced emotion seemed to come out of nowhere, it came with immediate insight into its origins. As neurosurgeon Henry Marsh says, "If one's in a bad mood, one might attribute it to having had an argument with somebody or worrying about something. But for all one knows, it might be also due to some neurochemical doing something for some reason."[2] You never know. For mindfulness purposes, it doesn't matter. What is more important is being present with emotions and processing them as they arise—now. If you see the emotion as a weather pattern passing through, you don't have to take it all so personally.

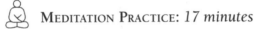

moods and foods

As long as our orientation is toward perfection or success, we will never learn about unconditional friendship with ourselves, nor will we find compassion.

—PEMA CHÖDRÖN

MEDITATION PRACTICE: *17 minutes*

DAY SEVENTEEN, *Meditation on Breath and Bodily Sensations*

If you are presently piling plenty of colorful plants on your plate, you are already at a better mood advantage. Research tells us that plant-based diets are associated with healthier mood states. The more fruits and vegetables people eat, the happier, less depressed, and more satisfied they are with their lives. Today, we'll focus on how, grounded in your biochemistry, eating more plants and eliminating animals and their products from your diet creates greater mental well-being and resilience.[1-2]

Plantified Plate = Mood Elevator Up

A recent study of nearly one thousand men and women examined the mood impact of obtaining dietary antioxidants. Antioxidants are health- and disease-protective bioactive chemical compounds produced by plants. In the study, those who ate three or more servings of fruits and vegetables a day reported significantly greater optimism than those who ate less.[3] Eating lots of veggies also bumps up the B vitamins in your diet, positively affecting mood states.[4]

Another recent, large-population, multi-wave study—taking place five times over the course of nine years—focused on the impact of fruit and vegetable intake on depression, anxiety, and mental health disorders. Results were consistent across all five waves: greater fruit and vegetable consumption was positively associated with reduced depression, less psychological distress, fewer mood and anxiety problems, and improved perceived mental health.[5]

Study after study corroborates. A large Swiss survey reported significant associations between higher fruit and vegetable consumption and reduced distress levels. People who ate less than the five-servings-a-day recommendation had a higher likelihood of reporting stress and anxiety than those who didn't.[6] A recent study on women's health from Australia followed over six thousand women. The findings? Reduced depression among women who simply ate more than two pieces of fruit a day. And the benefit increased when accompanied by higher intakes of vegetables.[7]

Eudaemonic Well-Being—Beyond Happy Moods

New research correlates eating fruit and vegetables with other markers of well-being beyond happiness and life satisfaction in what is called eudaemonic well-being. Eudaemonic well-being is characterized by feelings of engagement, meaning, purpose, curiosity, and creativity—all qualities we value for flourishing in daily life.[8]

Cut the Meat—Improve Your Mood

We get it—eating more plants boosts your mood. What if we look at it another way—*cutting out* the meat? How might that affect your state of mind? As it turns out, emotional resiliency and elevated mood states arise for more reasons than simply because you know you are doing the right thing. There's a deeper biochemical component that underpins well-being that comes with veganizing your plate.

According to research, reduced intake of animals and their products has mood benefits *in addition* to those that come with a robust daily intake of fruits and vegetables. Avoiding meat, fish, and poultry leads to more frequent reports of positive states of mind. And vegans report lower anxiety and less stress than omnivores.[9]

Our instincts tell us that the enormous stress and suffering experienced by animals in the conditions they face in the animal-agriculture industry cannot help but be passed along to whoever eats their bodies. We know that stress states that are part of the human experience—agitation, worry, fear, panic, grief, distress, sadness—inspire a corresponding biochemical reaction in our bodies. We also know that animals, as sentient beings, experience these same states. So what does that say about the eating of animals who experience extreme distress? Is the stress animals experience in the process of meat and dairy production passing along an infusion of disturbing biochemical compounds to the people who eat their bodies?

Research on this very topic has taken place. Not out of concern for the welfare of animals, as you might presume. Rather, concern over the quality and marketability of the meat itself has prompted such studies. The language used to advise meat production companies, such as "Stress before slaughter also affects the microbiological contamination in the live animal by influencing the meat quality, which may result in a more contaminated carcass," is more than alarming. Warnings of the effects on meat quality as a result of "great physical and psychological labor in clinically healthy animals" experienced in the farm-to-slaughter process—intended as quality control to the animal-product industry—underscores the stress and suffering perpetuated.[10] Is it possible that science is finally catching up with the centuries-old mindfulness practice tradition that advises a vegetarian/ vegan diet? That because every fiber of a slaughtered animal's body is vibrating with their experiences, eating that animal's body causes a negative, agitating effect on you?

Why Risk It?

Putting it all together, the Western diet—characterized by scanty consumption of plant foods, yet heavy on the animal products—is associated with increased risk of depression.[11] Depression is related to inflammation in the body. Arachidonic acid, found only in animal products, is a precursor to inflammation. Research shows that high intakes of arachidonic acid promote changes in the brain that can disturb mood.[12] Here's how it works. By eating chicken, eggs, and other animal products high in arachidonic acid, a series of chemical reactions is triggered in your body that results in inflammation. When inflammation reaches the brain, feelings of anxiety, stress, hopelessness, and depression follow.[13] No wonder people who avoid animal flesh and products report a happier, more positive mood.[14] And plant foods—to the rescue, once again—naturally *lower* inflammation due to their naturally high antioxidant content, antioxidants being one of nature's most powerful anti-inflammatory agents.

Nutrients provide the biological building blocks for neurotransmitters—the chemicals in your brain that deeply affect how you think and feel. When you aren't eating enough vitamins, minerals, antioxidants, polyphenols, and related nutrients found in plants—known in this context as neuronutrients—you can't make adequate mood-enhancing transmitters. These gems of plant nutrition, by the way, are the same goodies proved to be brain protective against Alzheimer's disease and other forms of dementia. Diets rich in the kind of saturated fats that are abundant in animal products—and deficient in antioxidants and vitamins—appear to promote the onset of the disease, whereas diets rich in plant-plentiful vitamins, antioxidants, and polyphenols suppress its onset.[15] All the colors plants bring to your plate are evidence of the nutrients your brain needs for better disposition. No wonder just seeing your luncheon salad makes your mood brighten.

Mindful Moment: Traditions

Historically, the mindfulness tradition embraces the precept of compassion toward all sentient beings and links meditation practice with compassion for animals. This includes abstaining from taking the lives of animals for consumption, releasing us from the negative mental states that come with it. It also underscores an aspiration for good-heartedness, care for yourself, and care for others.

Striving to act in ways that reduce the amount of suffering in the world, both for ourselves and for others, is a foundation of living mindfully. And mindfulness practice itself unearths compassion, naturally inspiring more conscious food choices, as Wendy Werneth, a vegan author and blogger, experienced:

> Two years ago, I finally brought my actions into line with my values and began living a life of compassion and non-violence. My only regret is that I didn't do it sooner. I hesitated for months, worried about all the ways I thought being vegan would make my life difficult. In reality, it has filled my life with joy, peace, and a sense of purpose.
>
> Through my meditation practice, I've gradually been training my mind to be present, to actually experience the current moment instead of constantly thinking about either the past or the future. By being in the moment when I'm eating, not only do I get to fully enjoy the eating experience, I'm also more aware of how full I am and of whether or not I really want to be eating.

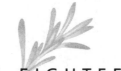

moods and mindfulness

Feel the rain on your skin
No one else can feel it for you
Only you can let it in

—NATASHA BEDINGFIELD, "Unwritten"

MEDITATION PRACTICE: *18 minutes*

DAY EIGHTEEN, *Moods; Meditation on Breath and Bodily Sensations*

Food is clearly a critical part of the mood equation. Yet what about day-to-day stresses that bring out our dark side, making moods plummet?

Until recently, it was believed that we all possessed a certain "mood set point" that stays fairly constant over the span of our lives. We now know there is a distinct relationship between your characteristic mood profile—your overall tendency to certain mood states over other moods—and which side of the prefrontal cortex of your brain is dominant. When the right side is more dominant, there is a correlation with higher rates of depression. When the left side prevails, the overall mood is happier. The good news? How you use your brain can affect which side is dominant.

When neuroscientists discovered that Tibetan monks, with decades of training in meditation and compassion practice under their belts, have higher left prefrontal cortex activation relative to hundreds of other people tested, the next question was obvious: Is this brain profile due to meditation practices, some other lifestyle factor, or an inherent quality in those who opt for the life of monkhood? To find out, they studied before-and-after brain imaging on participants in an eight-week mindfulness training. Researchers demonstrated that meditation for forty-five minutes daily for eight weeks was enough to increase activity in the left prefrontal cortex that corresponded to mood improvements, proving that mood "set points" can be altered.[1]

This is perhaps no more profoundly demonstrated than the way mindfulness impacts a familiar stress that we experience every day: our habit of getting mired in our thoughts. That maddening and tiresome playing of an event over and over in your mind that saps your energy and tanks your mood. Seduced by our own thoughts, unable to tear ourselves away yet wishing we could, sometimes it's as if we're addicted to thinking itself. Mindfulness training helps you out of this chronic mess by giving you a tool to leverage in ruminative moments, directly impacting brain activity as an antidote for negative moods.[2]

The Downside of Overthinking— and How Mindfulness Changes It

The habit of overthinking things, clinically referred to as *cognitive rumination*, hooks into habitual thought patterns—via specific brain pathways—that keep you caught up in stressful situations, amplifying sadness, anxiety, and just plain bad moods.[3] As we explored in Wandering Mind, Unhappy Mind (page 60), mindfulness practice puts dynamic tools of mood self-regulation in your hands.

Mood and emotion self-regulation via mindfulness is not to be confused with thought suppression ("I shouldn't be mad") or avoidance ("Don't think about it!") that magnify the problem.[4] Rather, with mindfulness, you direct your attention toward present-moment sensations in dedicated fashion. This delivers a new, nonthreatening focus for your attention that does not elicit brain activity associated with depression and sadness as does obsessive mental replay. Which, as we know, loops you into the default mode network.

The engagement of open, present-moment attention, such as you are practicing with meditation, activates brain pathways that allow you to respond with more objectivity. Instead of flying off the handle with a fired-up, conditioned reaction, with mindfulness you cultivate the ability to respond to situations with more rationality and equanimity.[5]

Case in point. A couple of days ago I was waiting at a stoplight on a country road. As the light turned green, I eased my foot off the brake and slowly started to accelerate. At about the same time, the driver in the car behind me, leaning on his horn, nearly crawled up the back of my car in apparent urgency to get moving faster than I was. There are three different ways I could have processed this experience: in research they are known as rumination, reappraisal, or mindfulness.

Rumination: I could have gotten all riled up and railed on about how impatient drivers are these days, and used some colorful language to express the angry reaction I could sense below the surface. I could have kept my thoughts focused on my evaluation of the situation, justified my own anger, and continued to scold the other driver in my mind. Now, we've all done this or been witness to this kind of reactivity to traffic impropriety. In the absence of emotion regulation, the effect is replaying the stressful situation, re-creating feelings of upset and negativity.

Reappraisal: In the case of reappraisal, the tone of evaluation shifts. While mentally noting that we all seem to be in such a hurry these days—and annoyed about it at that—I could have given the driver in question the benefit of the doubt. Maybe someone in the vehicle is about to deliver a baby. Perhaps there is some other emergency to which the driver is attending. Maybe they're just having a bad day. Even in this case of gracious reappraisal, however, attention is still repeatedly directed toward replaying the event. You keep recalling the stressor you are trying to defuse.

Mindfulness: With a mindfulness response, I could allow the stressful-event story to remain in the past and turn my attention to present-moment sensations. How does my body feel in reaction to what's happened? How do my hands feel on the driver's wheel? I could quickly scan my emotional centers for sensations. Is there a tightening in the chest, a lump in my throat? Can I feel an adrenaline rush? Are my thoughts racing? Thoughts can create an almost palpable pull to replay and dissect situations. Mindfulness training limits the need to manipulate emotions through evaluation—in an attempt to rationally control the situation—in favor of bringing acknowledgment and curiosity to present-moment experience. In this case, the offending driver, regardless of his true motivations, is left in the past where he or she can cause no further upset. And I avoid stimulating brain pathways that can conjure sadness, depression, and a bad mood.

My response in this situation was a short reappraisal before implementing mindfulness of sensation as described above. Not only did this deliver the benefits already mentioned, but I also avoided piling on stress that seeks release later. This is a play-by-play example of how mindfulness practice leads to reduced stress, increased happiness, and more skillful living.

When you get right down to it, isn't what we are really seeking, with all our aspirations, happiness? Whether we want a better job, a better house, or better health—what we really want is to be happy.

✿ Mindful Moment: Overthinking Diet

"Diet takes up 90 percent of my thinking time. Every day I pour over websites about plant-based and vegan eating, and it gets confusing and very tiresome. I get so turned around in my thinking sometimes. It seems like the harder I try the more setbacks I have. I long to not be so consumed by my diet!"

Janet, my client, had started to realize how much she overthinks dietary plans. She admitted she was spending hours each day debating food plans, fussing over what might help her lose weight the fastest. This resulted in massive better-diet burnout.

Continuing to hit the hammer on the nail over and over all day long doesn't get the bridge built. To move forward with greater ease and confidence, at some point it is necessary to disengage from all the dietary debate. It's a looping treadmill that keeps us locked in, sad, and doubting. Once we become aware, as Janet did, that we are hopelessly locked in this cycle, we have taken the first giant step toward disentangling ourselves from a painfully unproductive mental spiral.

Expanding nutritional knowledge has opened our eyes to the benefits of plant-centering our plates. Yet information overload has driven us to a preoccupation with the finer details. This distracts us from simply improving our choices. It fosters a disconnect from our internal awareness about such basics as hunger and fullness and it harbors a mistrust in our bodies. Our enjoyment of food has become riddled with anxiety and ambivalence, and guilt has replaced comfort when we indulge in tasty pleasures. How do we free ourselves from these habits of thinking and end the misery of getting sucked into the same vortex day after day?

During meditation, you are letting thoughts parade by. What would happen if you applied that same observational quality to the constant stream of thoughts about eating, diets, food plans, or weight loss that can, for some, haunt you all day? How can you become free from the obsession about your weight, your health, your food?

Begin by being observant as these thoughts present themselves to you during the day. Even if you initially follow them and get involved in their stories, start by identifying and naming these thinking events. You could quietly note them for how they are showing up: first "thinking," then "thinking about weight," or "dieting," "debating," or "obsessing." Even if at first you get caught up in them, you will start to build mindfulness about what is hijacking your thinking. From there, you can leverage your growing ability to simply not follow these thoughts. Have they ever really gotten you anywhere? Doubts will come up; that's part of the mind's job—and we should investigate things thoroughly to make sure we are making the best choice. But haven't you already done that?

Be aware that once you stop engaging in these ruminative debates, you may experience one or both of the following. You may feel a sense of loss, simply because this thinking loop is what you are used to. You may feel fear, for somehow we got the idea that if we stop thinking about our diet, or weight, or health, we'll fall down the failure elevator shaft. Actually, the opposite is true. Obsessive thinking, as we now know, leads to downer moods, cravings, and less likelihood that you'll follow through on a healthy plan.

I asked Janet, "Don't you really already know enough about plant-based nutrition to do what you need to do?"

With a big sigh of relief, she answered, "Yes!"

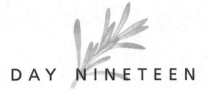

higher ground and mindfully navigating conversations

Mindfulness must be engaged. Once there is seeing there must be acting. Otherwise what is the use of seeing?

—THICH NHAT HANH

Meditation Practice: *19 minutes*

◁)) *Day Nineteen, Meditation on Breath and Bodily Sensations*

 "What a great title," Patti Breitman—longtime vegan, author, advocate, mindfulness meditator, and friend—commented as we sat down to have a chat over green drinks about *The Mindful Vegan*. These words were her immediate response to the name of the book. "It's almost redundant," she added.

Patti's right. By embracing vegan living, you are acting on your ethics mindfully, in a profound way. You are taking an active stand against the current norm that ignores the environmental crisis and reduces sentient beings, as all animals are, to things. Wherever you find yourself on the spectrum—from aspiring vegan to advocate to activist—you've moved to higher ground.

Yet sometimes it can feel as if you are swimming upstream, can't it? Every time you see animals listed as edibles on the menu—or a burger on a billboard, or a "happy chicken nuggets" commercial—you recognize how deeply embedded the problem is in our culture. As clear as it is to you that using animals as "products" must be halted—along with the pillaging of our planet that perpetuates the project—the stress and pain you feel can be profound. Johan Galtung, principle founder of the discipline of peace and conflict studies, said that the definition of violence is any "avoidable impairment of fundamental human needs."[1] It's time we broaden the definition to include all sentient beings. When you perceive the dairy case in the market as violence, the effect can be an overwhelming sense of urgency: things need to change—*now*!

We are mystified at how simply being present as a vegan at the table can provoke hostility, resistance, even accusations from others. You are probably not the first who has been called judgmental just because you brought veggie burgers to the office picnic or passed on the turkey at Thanksgiving. We can tell ourselves that this hostility has nothing to do with us and that it is merely projection by others. But it still stings and brings up feelings of defensiveness, frustration, and isolation.

To gain more insight into some of these challenges that you may be experiencing, today we'll take a glimpse into the meat culture and why it can be hard to bring others—friends, family, and coworkers—on board. Getting under the surface of this phenomenon can be of great help. You'll find out more about what can give rise to the resistance you experience—important information for everything from the playing field of daily living to the front lines of activism. And we'll underscore why your mindfulness practice—*inner* activism—is so important for vegan advocacy and activism of the outer kind.

The Meat Paradox

Everyone says they love animals. Most people don't enjoy the thought of harming or killing animals, and they instinctively rush in to free the wild bird from their cat's claws. Everyone wants to put an end to ivory poaching and to free Willy. So why do so many people pound down animal flesh—sometimes several times a day—and even criticize you for doing differently?

You don't have to look far to find examples of people holding on to their beliefs and practices in the face of overwhelming evidence to the contrary. This is no less true when it comes to people clinging to their ideas about what's for dinner. Meet the "meat paradox": when people like to eat meat but do not like to think of animals dying to provide it.

"If you scratch the surface, everybody seems to be a bit uncomfortable about eating meat," says Brock Bastian, a psychologist at the University of Melbourne in Australia, adding, "One of our most deeply and widely held moral concerns is to prevent harm."[2] Given our affection for "all creatures great and small," the idea of causing animals harm is at least a little disturbing. And the more someone likes animals while also eating meat, the more pronounced the conflict.

Yet people will do or say just about anything to defend their behaviors and avoid budging from the norm. This includes employing a variety of tactics to ease the discomfort resulting from the inner conflict—dissonance—of being an animal lover and an animal eater at the same time. This dissonance drives the modern meat industry's cage-free, free-range movement, providing a little guilt relief. It has given birth to the ethical meat-eating movement, a.k.a. "conscious omnivorism."[3]

According to cognitive dissonance theory, people alleviate this dissonance by altering one of the elements of the inconsistency: attitudes toward meat or attitudes toward animals. This dietary dissonance also creates a defensiveness in a way you might least expect. When a person's confidence in their current choices and habits (such as eating meat) is shaken, they become even *stronger* advocates for these same practices.[4] So though you may find it perplexing and infuriating, pushing harder for dietary change often only galvanizes that which you are advocating against. In other words, if someone is conflicted about what's on their plate, that can make you the number-one bad guy. Remember this next time someone goes over the top in coming down on your vegan plate in defense of their quarter pounder. They may well have unsettled emotions about it—and your presence, the reminder.

Research tells us that omnivores figure out lots of other ways to cope with cognitive dissonance to bring their beliefs and behavior in line.

This includes denying that animals used as food suffer. If the thought of eating meat and the misery and "unpleasantness" caused by the meat creates too much inner conflict, they may escape the conflict by seeing animals as unworthy and unfeeling. It conveniently shifts, in their minds, the animal's moral status.[5]

People can also be so identified with "the way things have always been" that considering uprooting long-held dietary practices creates deep resistance—overriding the dissonance. They might demonstrate denial that animals are killed in the process of meat production—reinforced by our euphemistic use of "beef" for cows or "pork" with pigs. Linguistic camouflage at its finest. Perceived behavioral change is another symptom. How many people have you met who claim they are vegetarian yet add that they eat fish? And in a related matter, people tenaciously cling to dietary practices because it is so bound up with their identity with a certain group.[6] It's the inclusion-in-the-clan phenomenon. Being identified with a social group has evolutionary roots: inclusion meant survival. Breaking out of this norm can feel unsettling not because of the food issue itself, but because it breaks with the norm.

Understanding this can give us insights into reluctance over dietary shifts, even in the face of strong evidence toward the positive aspects of change. So when you are eating tofu instead of turkey, it can trigger profound inner conflict and under-the-surface anxiety in your tablemates in a classic case of what is known as the beach ball effect, eloquently described by Will Tuttle in *The World Peace Diet* (Lantern Books, 2005):

> The vegan commitment to consciously minimize our cruelty to all animals is so revolutionary in its implications that it is often summarily dismissed because it triggers cognitive dissonance and deep anxiety...Like a ball being held under the water, our natural compassion wants to come bobbing up to the surface, so we must continually work to keep it repressed. The way we keep the ball of kindness and intelligence submerged is not only by practicing disconnecting, but also by the practice of nurturing some culturally induced objections to eating a plant-based diet, which we repeat to ourselves if the ball keeps rising.

The entire cognitive dissonance problem can come to a head at family affairs or social occasions where both omnivores and vegans or vegetarians are present. Here, the presence of people with differing dietary practices shines a big spotlight on the elephant in the room—the meat paradox. The inner discomfort people experience explains the awkward feelings at the dinner table. Things can even get tense between people who say they are vegan or vegetarian for ethical reasons and those who do so for health reasons, as individuals jockey into positions of judgment. [7]

While rationalizing enables omnivores to continue eating as they do, the good news is that eating animal products has increasingly come under public scrutiny and become socially subject to criticism. And although meat eating is still the norm in most countries, many people, including meat eaters themselves, believe that vegetarianism is a morally admirable practice for which vegetarians deserve credit. So the norm has started to shift.[8]

You: The Face of Vegan Living

Mindful of the meat paradox climate, how can you best be present to make a difference? The most immediate influence you can be in the hearts and minds of others is to exemplify the change you want to see. This doesn't mean being perfect or having the healthiest body in the county. It is rather on the level of presence. This is the predominant current thinking for effective vegan advocacy, and it extends to those times when you are actively and openly advocating for vegan living.[9] People respond more to your presence and how you treat them, how you listen to them, and how consistent you are than to what you say. It is your heart, clarity, centeredness, and compassion with which people will connect.

People experience *you* more than the words that come out of your mouth. What are you saying with your voice, your manner, your presence? Do you think they are more likely to consider the change you stand for if you are constantly stressed out, hostile, and judgmental? If your demeanor is dour and disheveled? If you make vegan living look hard, inconvenient, or devoid of tasty food? Or are they more likely to venture into vegan living if they see it modeled well in your happiness, patience, friendliness, and kindness? If they see that you, too, are aspiring to something—and leave perfectionism at the door? That your food is appealing, delicious, and satisfying on all fronts?

If you do or say something with a certain feeling tone, the results are going to carry that same flavor. And how you respond will have a feedback loop effect—on your own life as well as that of others. Think back to a point in time when you were influenced to move away from a certain long-held belief or toward doing something in a new way—maybe even to the idea of becoming vegan. Who was the person that influenced you to make a change? What was it about them that opened your heart, that caused you to listen? Was it more about who they were, and how they were toward you, than what they said? A combination of factors?

The practice of mindfulness will help you create a clearer inner personal environment for vegan living by allying your strong personal conviction with nonreactivity, compassion, and kindness. This can dramatically impact your influence in the world, let alone your personal happiness. If your current way of navigating conversations about food choices and other reaches of vegan living is delivering good results and growing your sphere of influence along with your own happiness, peace, and ease of living, by all means carry on. But if you are experiencing anxiety, stress, or agitation and find it difficult to disentangle inner and outer conflict while navigating these conversations, practicing and applying mindfulness to your encounters can open the door to a better way. After all, how can we expect to foster peace and harmony in anyone else if we are not experiencing them ourselves?

Navigating Conversations

No one feels good after being scolded; generally, people recoil and become angry, defensive, or stubborn. To succeed in freeing people to express compassion—to open their hearts and minds, letting the beach ball rise to the surface and unleash them from the meat paradox—our interactions must be rooted in empathy for and understanding of the uncomfortable inner conflict they may be facing. This is done through working with their motivations, fears, desires, and shortcomings—not through shame and hostility. Whether you receive praise or blame in these interactions is out of your hands. You have to let go of having control over what the outcome or response to your sharing will be, in favor of being at peace with your own integrity and knowing that the power of intention is the most important factor in everything you do.

Your mindfulness practice will help you get out of brain lock with set patterns so you can respond to conflict and difficult situations with more finesse. It teaches you how to live more aligned with the ethical life to which you aspire—being kind in your works and your speech, being rooted in nonviolence, doing everything you can to not cause more violence in your personal interactions. The very awareness and inner peace you cultivate with mindfulness can touch and awaken the same in others.

Mindfulness of Emotion in Action

When speaking or dealing with others, see if you can become aware of any reactivity within you. You can sense it in your body—the feeling of a racing energy or righteousness—and how it pulls you away from being present, away from a place of confidence and inner connectivity. Any point in the process in which you can notice reactivity is helpful. Sometimes you are with a veg-friendly crowd that is open and receptive. When, on the other hand, you have difficult conversations, reactivity is what you are most likely encountering. By adding your own reactivity to the mix, hostility is a likely outcome.

Being Prepared

Mindfulness practice will help you more peacefully thrive amid and more effectively navigate conversations. It edifies your ability to be present with these challenges with greater ease—due to the equanimity, resiliency, and compassion you cultivate with your practice.

Equanimity

Equanimity is a state of balance and poise. It is often confused with withdrawal or hesitation. But equanimity in our dealings with others is far from indifference or passivity, as such states of disconnection are actually subtle forms of hostility toward our experience.[10] Equanimity is rather the ability to be balanced and present, which always leads to better communications. In the context of mindfulness practice, equanimity means being fully connected with what is going on without being caught up in the drama of whatever is unfolding. It is the ability to stand firm yet without rigidity. While mindfulness emphasizes your ability to remain consciously aware of what is happening in the field of your experience, equanimity allows your awareness to be even and less biased. It is what invites the space to open up between an event, internal or external, and reactivity.

There is nothing wrong with the anger or fear that you may feel arising in yourself when in conversations about food choice. In these situations you can feel as if you have to fight like mad to control your emotions. With mindfulness, however, you have a new tool with which to navigate these feelings so that they do not hijack your temperament, crippling your ability to reach another heart. In mindfulness practice, equanimity has been called "radiant calm of mind" or "spacious stillness of heart." Research even suggests that equanimity captures "potentially the most important psychological element in the improvement of our well-being."[11] Each day, in your formal mindfulness practice as you patiently return to anchor, let go of wandering thoughts, and survey sensations with calm and composure, you are directly practicing the same equanimity that is your ally in these and every life situation.

When you notice these emotions arising—which you are learning how to do with mindfulness practice—rather than reacting to them, or avoiding, resisting, or denying them, first cultivate awareness of them. Turn your inner lens to staying present with the sensations of emotions as they come up, just as you practice every day in your meditation, taking away their power to grab a hold of and run away with your attention, well-being, and everything else. This delivers more inner calm, connectivity, and confidence. You can then better proceed with strong conversation born of conviction, spoken from a state of openness and compassion. It doesn't mean you always get it right—keep aspiration and intention as your companions. For the beginning meditator confronted with an emotionally charged situation, equanimity can be even more fleeting. It will come with practice.

Resiliency

Resiliency is your bounce-back ability. It is the capacity to withstand stress and hardship. You enhance resiliency through regular mindfulness practice, which shifts you from being caught up in the drama or "stories" surrounding an event to noticing your experience with kind attention.

This practice causes a shift in your neural pathways—out of your reactive, fear-based emotional processing into your higher brain structures of reasoning and executive function. This strengthens a more regulated emotional process—granting you the ability to better engage your inner resources for appropriate response. This is enormously helpful in navigating conversations, especially about something as potentially charged as diet. Cultivating a positive view of yourself helps maintain resiliency. Learn to listen to your instincts and needs; get support and accept help when you need it.

Compassion

We are animals, too. What of compassion for yourself? Once we understand that a sustainable, thriving vegan lifestyle is fundamental not only to our personal peace and happiness but to the entire movement, maybe we'll make some traction in self-care. Doing what you can do to reduce stress and increase resiliency isn't just a good idea; it's imperative. The minutes that you carve out each day for mindfulness practice are a vital investment in your personal well-being that pay off big-time in dividends to the vegan community at large. Simply by making you more connected, grounded, and . . . well, cared for.

Self-compassion isn't self-pity. It is warmth, care, concern, and good wishes—just as the compassion you have for other beings. It's being patient with your progress. Become aware of your needs: for restorative time, for healthy food, for physical exercise, for love and laughter. These give you more resiliency, too. The compassion and kindness you extend to yourself are of such importance that we will dive even deeper into it in tomorrow's lesson, Cultivating Kindness and Compassion.

Listening and Speaking with Mindfulness

Mindfulness is a quality that allows you to listen and speak with kindness and equanimity as a natural outgrowth. Here are some of the ways that you can bring them forward into your conversations, interpersonal relationships—even presentations, should the opportunity arise.

Listening

We all sense the difference when someone genuinely listens to us without lying in wait until they can make their point. Likewise, when we listen to someone else without the charged atmosphere of agenda, we both notice the difference. Let go of agenda and listen with a clear, nonjudgmental attitude. I know this can be hard. It seems all day we are making judgment calls, especially regarding something as fundamental as the values we hold so dear. But the first step toward being heard is to listen.

When in a conversation, mindfully notice any thoughts or judgments that haven't taken up residence in your mind. This includes making assumptions about what the other person is about to say and judgments about the person with whom you are speaking. Once aware of these appraisals, you are better able to let go of them—just as you have been practicing letting go of thoughts during mindfulness practice. This creates a safer environment for open conversation. Mindfully maintain eye contact, showing your interest, courtesy, and attention. Become aware of how any agenda you may have started to appear. As you become more practiced in mindfulness of bodily sensations, you will be able to feel these thoughts arising in your body as tension or resistance.

Notice any judgment you feel toward the person with whom you are talking, and what they are saying. You will notice that you probably have a preconceived notion of what they are about to say—even who they are. Once aware of the judgment, you are better able to let it go.

You may be feeling that by listening with a nonjudgmental attitude you are somehow condoning that which you are seeking to change. But it doesn't work that way. If you speak from the heart with a balanced mind, your confidence and kindness are what people hear.

Speaking and the Self-Affirmation Theory

When it comes to navigating these conversations, remember—people who may be waffling on an issue tend to galvanize their stance when it is threatened, even though they may feel uncertain of their position. Interestingly, there's more to the story. Research tells us that these galvanizing effects are lessened when people experience self-affirmation of their important personal values before being presented with ideas contrary to their current, though somewhat softened, stance. Apparently, if self-esteem is bolstered in advance of receiving information that conflicts with someone's identity, it has a way of offsetting perceived threat and makes people more likely to be open-minded. This is known as the self-affirmation theory, which loops back to the fact that people are motivated to maintain integrity of self-identity. When acknowledged and supported, we are less likely to be resistant to new ideas. This can be critical to our communications with others about vegan living—and all our other life encounters, too.[12]

This probably comes as no surprise to you if you've ever been in debate about food choice. Even if you are armed with all the facts about the animals, health, and the environment, you are bringing to light flaws within a concept that may be central to someone else's self-identity. In light of the need people have to maintain their integrity, a strong reaction is normal and makes perfect sense. The hope underlying their strengthened position is that they will be able to convince you to switch to their side. This hooks back into the clan phenomenon—there's safety in numbers. If you believe as they do, it lessens any inner conflict they may be feeling.

So what is the big takeaway from these studies? Simply going into a debate about vegan living armed with the artillery of logic and statistics will probably not work in the way you are certain or hopeful that it will. Whoever is in your virtual line of fire will fall back behind the cognitive dissonance barricade. Instead of viewing others as someone with whom you disagree, see them as a human. Take the time to get to know them, what is important to them, something about them that you can genuinely appreciate. Without such a connection, it's likely the conflict will escalate as they up their fervor.

Building an armed battleground does not create a landscape of respect and connection. Regular mindfulness practice creates new pathways in your mind that bring you back to the clarity and openness of presence. This helps keep you more grounded and better equipped to navigate the anxiety and stress these conversations can present.

Mindful Moment: Timing

While speaking up and speaking out make a difference, timing can be just as important as presentation. When approaching a conversation, make a decision about whether or not this is the time to engage in the topic. Has someone asked you a specific question regarding diet and sincerely expressed a desire to find out more? Have they seen how you consistently make certain choices? Are they impressed by the lifestyle confidence and resiliency you seem to embody most of the time and want to find out more about that? Do they have a health issue and thought you might be a good resource? Were they just alerted to the startling impact that animal agriculture has on the environment and want to ask you for more information? Are they simply interested in what you have brought to eat for lunch—or want the recipe for the spectacular enchilada pie you brought to the potluck?

The entry points for conversation about vegan living go on and on. This short list just gives you an idea of all the different pathways there are to becoming vegan. Can you answer from authentic experience, in a way that doesn't express judgment or condescension to the other person? And consider your own vulnerability. Just because you meditated this morning doesn't mean you're a tower of strength and composure. If you are feeling vulnerable, consider this in your conversation, and think about compassionately removing yourself from sensitive parts of the conversation until a better time.

For additional support in navigating these conversations, *Why We Love Dogs, Eat Pigs, and Wear Cows* by Melanie Joy, as well as videos and other information provided at carnism.org—which discuss dealing with communication and relationship issues at length—deliver enormous insight and provide valuable tips.

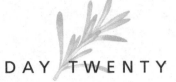

cultivating kindness and compassion

*The most effective people are those that are most sustained.
When we are more inner connected, not only are we better
ambassadors, but we have more energy, make better choices,
and act more effectively. Mindfulness reflects the core values of
the vegan movement—by bringing compassion to yourself.*

—MELANIE JOY, PhD

MEDITATION PRACTICE: *20 minutes*

DAY TWENTY, *Loving Kindness Meditation*

   The disturbing reality surrounding various forms of animal exploitation, and the environmental degradation caused by animal agriculture, can be tough to bear. Vegan advocates and activists often feel that their efforts for change are not making enough difference. This can lead to frustration and burnout, making people susceptible to what is known as compassion fatigue.

"The beauty of what you are doing is you have a recipe that can be applied to everything," Melanie Joy, a sustainable activism expert, said to me when we met to talk about *The Mindful Vegan*. Vegans often wonder if they are doing enough for the vegan cause if they aren't feeling a constant sense of urgency and outrage. Yet people need to give *themselves* permission to relate to themselves with the same compassion they do to the animals.

"The most effective people," Melanie said, "are those who are most sustained by practicing taking care of their own needs. If we look and feel exhausted, angry, and deprived—in overwhelm and despair—then other people are not going to be as likely to want to become part of this movement. Mindfulness reflects the core values of the movement. We are animals, too. We practice compassion for the animals—what of compassion for ourselves?"

In the scope of mindfulness tradition is a form of meditation called loving kindness. Loving-kindness meditation involves direct well-wishing toward not only others but also ourselves. Perceive "mindfulness" as also "heartfulness," and you come closer to the true nature of this practice. Research shows that loving-kindness meditation promotes compassion for oneself as well as others, diminishing stress, social anxiety, and depression while enhancing positive mental states. This produces increased mindfulness, purpose in life, and life satisfaction.[1]

Today we'll look at why cultivating kindness and compassion toward yourself plays such an important part in your own well-being and resiliency and why "compassion satisfaction" is essential for offsetting compassion fatigue. We'll also learn a simple loving-kindness meditation.

Cultivating Compassion

The compassion you bring to your mindfulness practice reflects how you are with yourself outside of practice, how you are with others, and how you are in the world.

Paying Attention to How You Pay Attention

At your next sitting practice, investigate the attitude that you bring specifically to paying attention. What is the feeling tone you experience at the moment of remindfulness—that precise instant you realize that you've been lost in thought? What are the qualities of the way in which you bring your attention back?

How you are with yourself at this very moment gives you a lot of information about the kindness and compassion you hold for *you*. Maybe you are just matter of fact about it and come back to anchor like a GPS reroute. Perhaps you detect negative reactivity at the point of remindfulness, possibly reflected in negative self-talk. Do you feel exasperated or impatient? Do you admonish, blame, judge? Or do you react with "Oh, there I go again"; "How silly of me"; "How frustrating"—or even feelings of guilt? You may start to become aware of how these same reactions show up in the rest of your day, outside of formal practice, as admonishment or judgment toward yourself in other situations. This is one of the ways mindfulness forges a path to seeing your patterns and yourself as you really are—the first stride into change.

Your influence for creating a world of kindness and compassion for others is proportionate to how you extend these very qualities toward yourself. If you are impatient with and disparaging of yourself, then that is possibly the attitude with which you deal with others.

By cultivating the same compassion and kindness for yourself that you want to see in the world, it will proliferate in your life, your home, and your communications beyond. Along with clarifying our intentions to the best of our abilities, it allows our minds to become clearer and brighter. From this place of clarity, we can help others more effectively. This is the value of practicing kindness during meditation, and central to mindfulness meditation in the first place.

Negative reactions to wandering mind can be rewired. The moment you notice it, be willing to be present with it. Then, gently open up a space around it, letting in patience, understanding, and kindness for yourself.

Loving-Kindness Meditation

The longtime tradition of what is known as loving-kindness meditation nurtures kindness and compassion toward—and beyond—yourself. Historically, people who have the strongest loving-kindness meditation practice tend to do better at getting through life's ebbs and flows. This underscores why it is important that you pay attention not just to the present moment experiences, but also to the qualities of *how* you pay attention.

Loving-kindness meditation uses words and feelings to awaken compassion and friendliness toward yourself and others. As you mentally speak each phrase, you are expressing an intention, cultivating a heart of kindness. Not to be confused with affirmations, a technique of repeating phrases over and over to bring about an outcome, a loving-kindness phrase is a wish for something that is universally desirable. These phrases begin with "May you..." or "May I..." or "May all..." Affirmations can clash, sometimes cruelly, with reality. In contrast, a loving-kindness phrase is something you can connect with even when what you are evoking feels far from your present experience.[2]

My personal practice is to take the last few minutes of each formal meditation to practice loving-kindness meditation. It helps set an intention to be more mindful throughout the day. Though there are a few variations on the theme, this is the one that has the most meaning and benefit for me. You are welcome to borrow it, massage it to give it more personal meaning, or come up with your own. Quietly, mentally to myself, I usually close my formal sitting with the following phrases:

May I be happy, may I be healthy, may I be safe.
May I be more loving and kind.
May my life be filled with greater ease.
May my life be filled with greater joy.
May my life be filled with greater happiness.
May my life be filled with greater peace.

I will then repeat these phrases with someone else in mind—a family member, a friend, sometimes gatherings and groups, and sometimes for people whom I find difficult. I simply replace the word *I* with the word *you* while keeping the person or place in my heart.

May you be happy, may you be healthy, may you be safe.
May you be more loving and kind.
May your life be filled with greater ease.
May your life be filled with greater joy.
May your life be filled with greater happiness.
May your life be filled with greater peace.

Traditionally, this meditation can progress to "May all...," making the wish for well-being even broader. It's possible that this meditation may feel mechanical or awkward to you. It may even bring up feelings that are quite the opposite of loving kindness, such as irritation or anger. It may seem contrived or not genuine. Or that you are putting too much attention on yourself.

Admittedly, I didn't take to loving-kindness meditation right away. I felt there was an artifice about it, and initially, I couldn't tease it apart from what I knew about affirmations. But after some time, and once the benefits of mindfulness practice became so clear, I thought, gee, if the basics are delivering so well, maybe there is something to this loving-kindness practice after all. What I found was that it did have a bleed-over effect into increasing patience and kindness toward myself, along with greater happiness and joy. From there, my awareness grew around how I react to others and to situations that arise throughout the day—to life itself. So if you don't take to the idea of loving-kindness meditation right away, no worries. As always, should this be your experience, patiently receive whatever arises the best you can in a spirit of kindness.[3] You can always revisit the idea later if you like. At the same time, you may find it is just the thing to create more benevolence around your own practice. You can reverse the order and express loving kindness toward another before yourself, or add yourself at another time. Kindness and patience are the important thing.

The Second-Arrow Effect

One of the most powerful lessons in mindfulness tradition—when it comes to loving kindness—is what is known as the second-arrow effect. It goes something like this: Whenever we suffer a setback or disappointment, the actual misfortune is the first arrow. The second arrow is the one we ourselves send *after* the first. It is our reaction to the first, unfortunate event. It represents the manner in which we react emotionally. For example, let's say a friend makes a hurtful comment to you—first arrow. The sinking feeling in your heart, the cofactors of sadness and perhaps a little anger, are the second arrow. Later, you replay the scene in your mind, over and over. How could she say that to me? What was he thinking? Third arrow. Then resentment is layered in. Arrow number four. As the evening arrives, you wrestle with what to do next. Should I confront her? Is he oblivious and I need to let him know how wrong he was? Next arrow. By ten o'clock that night you find yourself scraping the bottom of a big bowl of ice cream, replaying the comment in your mind. Not long after that, you kick yourself for eating too much ice cream. How many arrows are we up to now?

Or, you arrive home from an afternoon of errands and much to your annoyance your significant other has—*again*—left their dishes in the sink. The dishwasher is just inches away, for cripes' sake. Frustration and anger can quickly rise in reaction. You start to conjure up how to make more of an impression with your dishes-in-the-sink lecture next time. The dishes are actually just a condition. No one was hurt and the sky didn't fall. It was just a discourtesy. Or maybe there is some other explanation—the dishwasher isn't working, or there was an emergency that needed immediate tending to. Maybe not.

The dishes in the sink are the first arrow. Do you really have to get upset? You could just move the dishes to the dishwasher, or talk with your spouse calmly about it. Sometimes I manage to handle situations like this with equanimity. But I'm not a paragon of virtue and can fly off the handle just like the next person—it's just that it happens less often, which is nice. But if it does happen, here comes the second arrow (anger and frustration) followed by a third arrow (self-righteousness over being mad about the dishes), occasionally a fourth arrow (taking it personally) . . . and sometimes a few more. The second-arrow suffering is well under way, along with a few of her sisters coming along for the ride. And now it's in your body as the nervous system scrambles into play, firing up all your stress cylinders. These reactions don't simply vanish, either. They leave a residue of tension that accumulates in your body, where they are held only to play back later with discomfort, agitation, and other disquieting states. You quickly spiral into the default mode network of rumination, contributing to the rise of anxiety, stress, reactivity—and potentially activating network cohorts such as cravings and sadness. You hand your well-being over to whether an experience is to your liking.

There is a way to interrupt these cycles of destructive impulses. Once you become more awakened to how you heap misery and stress upon yourself via the second-arrow effect, you open the door to creating a different experience. When you are not caught up in reacting to a situation, you are able to be more present with an artful response that is unique to each circumstance—including the dishes in the sink. You unpack the ability to navigate the potentially irritating things that come up several times a day. Mindfulness provides new territory between what happens and your response to it—will you react impulsively or with wisdom?

The first arrow is the initial event itself. The second arrow is the one you shoot into yourself. This arrow is optional. You can add to the initial pain in a contracted, angry, rigid, frightened state of mind. Or you can learn to experience the same event with less reactivity, identification, and aversion—with a more relaxed and compassionate heart—and take more skillful action. You can start to have some impact on how many arrows make their way into your back.

Implementing RAIN (page 134) is your ally for offsetting the barrage of an increasing number of arrows.

Combating Compassion Fatigue

Compassion fatigue is a recognized state that can be experienced by those helping others in distress. It is characterized by extreme tension and preoccupation with the suffering of those you are helping to the degree that it is traumatizing. Vegan activists and advocates may recognize the feeling. If accompanied by poor self-care and extreme personal sacrifice in the process of helping, compassion fatigue can lead to symptoms similar to posttraumatic stress disorder. You can become compassion fatigued either through helping or by the empathetic distress that providing support can cause—most likely both.

There is a restorative antidote—compassion *satisfaction*. "People get fatigued by caring, in the absence of sensing compassion satisfaction, if it is not held in a bigger container of 'I know what I can do, I am supported in doing that work, and I see the benefits of my giving, or helping, or responding,'" says Kelly McGonigal, PhD, of the Stanford Center of Compassion and Altruism, describing some of the qualities of compassion satisfaction.

There are limits to how one human can skillfully respond, and recognizing the need for the restorative qualities that compassion satisfaction brings is critical. Compassion burnout is a signal to reengage with your resources and invest in self-care. This includes recognizing your contribution, seeing how your actions have made a difference, being connected to a community that is working to relieve the same suffering as you, and mindfulness training.[4]

🪷 Mindful Moment: Self-Care

Some years ago, in addition to being a partner, parent, activist, event planner, and a writer, I found myself caregiver for my mother, who had developed early onset Alzheimer's. I felt nearly crushed by the indescribable grief along with the weight of all my responsibilities, and began to see my own health deteriorate. I felt like I was running on fumes—like when you're driving and your gas gauge is on empty but you have no opportunity to refuel. You have to keep driving it in the desperate hopes that you will find a station in time. This was how I felt all the time—burnt out, stressed, constantly worried, overwhelmed—without a refueling station in sight. It began to manifest as chronic insomnia, digestive upset, and generally feeling depleted all the time. I was running myself into the ground.

Thankfully, I had a conversation with a friend that turned everything around. She told me how vital it was that I prioritize my health and well-being. I'd already heard this a million times by well-meaning people and at first, the words just scattered like dry leaves. I think my friend could tell that

I wasn't really hearing her. She said, "If you don't care for yourself, you cannot care for anyone else." I told her that she was right, and that I would take better care of myself so I could be a better caregiver. Then she said something that resonated with me in a way that nothing had until that point. She said, "Okay, listen to me. You have to take care of yourself for yourself because you deserve it. No other reasons are necessary. You deserve kindness, too."

Many times, those of us who advocate on behalf of others think that we are selfish and weak for emphasizing self-care. We have guilt, self-contempt and delusions of invulnerability that keep us from being our own advocates. If you can't be kind to yourself, though, I would question how kind you are being to others. How much are you secretly keeping score? How much of your care giving is less about compassion and more about your ego or martyrdom? How much to prove that you're a good person? These are all questions that I had to honestly ask myself.

In that moment with my friend, I learned that being mindful of self-care was essential to my evolution as someone who is an advocate and who claims to be compassionate. I learned that if I took thirty minutes to exercise, the world wouldn't collapse. I learned if I asked relatives to visit with my mother so my husband and I could see a movie, they were glad to help. I learned that taking a bath, being more forgiving of myself, and taking an hour to go to the library and pick up some great books helped me to become a less miserly person who was getting comfortable in her victim status. I meditate for ten minutes every morning after sun salutations. It's not going to break any meditation records, but it works for me. Most important, recognizing, speaking to and taking care of my needs meant that I was showing up for myself as a compassionate, loving person who excludes no one. As my friend said to me, if for no other reason, be kind to yourself because you deserve kindness.[5]

—Marla Rose, cofounder of Veganstreetmedia.com

DAY TWENTY-ONE

attractivism

In what ways—by how we treat ourselves and react to others—
are we unwittingly multiplying the dynamics of that which we
are attempting to correct?

—OREN JAY SOFER, meditation teacher

MEDITATION PRACTICE: *21 minutes*

DAY TWENTY-ONE, *Meditation on Breath and Bodily Sensations*

As much as vegan living is taught, more often it is caught. Focusing on the positive aspects of vegan living and all the goods it brings to the table creates an activism that opens hearts to new reaches of compassion. Activism becomes attractivism: the effects can reach across philosophical differences and draw us closer together through the common ground of kindness.

Here is the story of how Karenna, vegan activist and creator of VeganGreen.org, demonstrated many of the qualities—care, kindness, and presence—that we have been discussing in the last two days. Karenna's unlikely friendship with a dairy farmer led to her being able to rescue Angel, a dairy cow destined for slaughter. Her sincere curiosity and interest in the farmer and his work is a great example of the self-affirmation theory.

Karenna: Attractivism in Action

One day not long ago, Karenna was driving home through the hills of Northern California when she passed a small dairy farm. Curious to see how a small dairy farm operated, she pulled over and asked the owner if she might take a look around.

"He was very friendly," Karenna told me—I suspect largely because Karenna presented as kind, curious, and friendly herself. He did not ask Karenna about why she wanted to see the ranch. He showed her the grounds and left her to explore on her own. An old-school farmer, the dairyman was retiring after seventy years.

A year later, passing through the same area, Karenna noticed that the farm had closed down. She spoke with the owner again. He had closed the family business and sold all his cows to another dairy. But he did have one young calf left, whom he was keeping in an outdoor pen. Karenna was introduced to Angel—not her name at the time, because, as the old farmer said, "We can't get to know them like that." His plan was to keep Angel another few months before she was grown enough to bring a good price at auction.

Right away, Karenna offered to take Angel off his hands. The word *rescue* had come up in previous conversations and created some resistance from the farmer. Karenna, sensitive to this, softened her language from *rescue* to *adopt*. That made all the difference. It took three more visits to the farm, where Karenna repeatedly offered to adopt the young cow, for the farmer to be convinced to turn young Angel over to a different fate. Karenna had found a specific home for Angel at Rancho Compasión, a nonprofit farm-animal sanctuary about an hour away. The farmer finally relinquished Angel, and Karenna paid him the amount that Angel may have brought at an auction.

The story of Karenna and Angel points out something we can all learn from. As outraged as we may feel at finding someone like Angel nameless and penned in a dirty enclosure in the back of a barn, if we come out with fingers shaking and accusations blazing, we create more distance and hostility than understanding and connection. Karenna demonstrated presence by developing a relationship with the farmer through repeated visits. She shared her own experiences growing up with a dad who hunted. She related to the farmer on his own terms and spoke to him without judgment or blame. As a result of the encounter with Karenna, the farmer had an experience of meeting someone who cares about animals and their welfare, about him and his work—which together formed a positive resolution for Angel's future. Meeting others with patience and kindness goes further to change hearts than being harshly judgmental and militant.

Karenna, whose work necessarily involves reviewing footage of inhumanity and injustices to animals on a daily basis, has also realized how critical it is to keep a daily practice to manage the stresses of activism. This is essential for her own well-being and to keep her more grounded and centered in conversations and interactions around compassion for animals.

As a result of Karenna befriending the farmer in such kind fashion, an animal was spared misery. Sometimes activism takes the form of reaching across the aisle and showing compassion toward humans, too— not just attacking them because they don't think like us. This farmer kept his cows until old age because he'd become attached to them. He thought he was feeding America, because that was all he knew.

"Had he met an in-your-face strident vegan activist rather than Karenna," said Rancho Compasión cofounder Miyoko Schinner, "Angel wouldn't be with us today."[1]

✿ Mindful Moment: What's Important?

What my practice has certainly taught me is to ask before interactions of any kind: Is this going to cause harm to myself or others? What that leads to is noticing that my compassion now extends to people as well as to animals. I do find that I am less judgmental. Or when I find myself judging another, I'm aware of it and can see that it's not helpful. Joanna Macy, one of my teachers and a respected voice in movements for peace, justice, and ecology, taught me that it's more important to connect heart-to-heart than to try to change someone's mind. So I'm more apt to talk with people without mentioning my veganism. I do mention it if anything makes me think to—and a lot does make me think to—but for the most part, I don't make it the "lead" in any conversation. If others ask, I'm still fiercely advocating for veganism. And my advocacy work with Dharma Voices for Animals is helping push for vegan policies at retreat centers. But personally, I find that angst, fretting, and pushy advocacy don't further the cause.

—Patti Breitman, cofounder, Dharma Voices for Animals

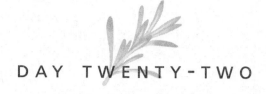

DAY TWENTY-TWO

spectrum of mindfulness practices

The best way out is always through.

—ROBERT FROST

MEDITATION PRACTICE: *22 minutes*

DAY TWENTY-TWO, *Meditation on Breath and Bodily Sensations*

In the early hours just after midnight today, we discovered a fox on the deck outside our house. He was busily nibbling on the wild birdseed we scatter daily for the birds and squirrels. Constantly lifting his head, he would turn his sensory focus from one side to the other as he listened carefully for every sound and watched closely for every single movement in the dark. I'm not sure if there is a fox equivalent of a default mode network, but if there is, I'm pretty sure it vacillates between attentive alertness and more attentive alertness.

Fox survival, much like that of every other being in the wild, depends on this kind of focused attention. Thank goodness we need not be so vigilant all the time. Yet the fox taught me something important. When I got up for practice a few hours later, as I settled into meditation, I thought of the fox and what I could learn from him. How could I bring the qualities of attentive alertness to my practice this morning? His focus on the food was an anchor point. At the same time, he was mindful of sounds and sights that presented themselves, which he would investigate with curiosity. When sights and sounds became less compelling, he went right back to anchor—the food.

There is a variation of the practices you have learned to date that is not unlike what the fox does—minus the edge of anxiety he must maintain for his survival—called choiceless awareness meditation. Let's take a quick look back at our practice and see how to bring choiceless awareness, along with the lesson from the fox, into play. From there, we'll continue along the spectrum of mindfulness practices and introduce open monitoring meditation.

Spectrum of Mindfulness Practices

Thus far, in formal meditation, you have been practicing *focused awareness* meditation. With focused awareness, you narrow your attention to a single object or event that you have chosen—the feelings of the breath or bodily sensations. Through this process you develop concentration, an important foundation of mindfulness meditation. The steadying awareness you experience helps move you away from reactivity and rumination into more presence of mind. Through this process you build the skills of self-regulation and cultivate a particular orientation to your experience—kindness, self-compassion, and patience—that helps tame the busy mind. This makes your capacity for mindfulness more available to you during the day, outside of formal practice.[1]

Choiceless Awareness Meditation

Choiceless awareness meditation also utilizes anchor. The difference is, while inhabiting the same awareness that you have been cultivating, you now let the object of anchor choose *you*.

Actually, you briefly encountered choiceless awareness on day two when you expanded your attention from the feeling of the breath to awareness of other sensations throughout your body. You start, as has been your practice, with meditation on the breath as anchor. Once your attention is gathered, you expand awareness to the body as a whole—to include bodily sensations, sounds, and emotions. When an element from any of these domains arises, strong enough to pull your attention from the breath, then this becomes your new anchor. It might be a sound or the sudden awareness of the feeling of an emotion, such as sadness, excitement, or anxiety. It might be a bodily sensation that seems unrelated to emotion.

Whatever arises, you stay with the new experience, letting go of analysis or getting involved in the story surrounding it—just as always with meditation on bodily sensations. When something else comes to your attention, then *that* becomes your anchor until the next thing comes along. If the sensation vanishes before another arises to pull your attention, simply reanchor at the feeling of the breath. There is no need to look for anything, or have any sense that something is wrong, if nothing arises. Simply be present with whatever is showing up, with curiosity and an open heart. Like the lesson of the fox, the idea is to let the phenomenon with the strongest presence choose you. It's more like an open dance card. And if nothing in particular presents itself, you stay with the feeling of the breath as anchor.

If at any point choiceless awareness feels overwhelming, distracting, or confusing, you return to the breath. Or you can let go of the idea of choiceless awareness altogether until a later date, when you feel more practiced with the breath and bodily sensations as anchor. The drawback of choiceless awareness is that you can miss the subtler stuff—only the stronger sensations jump out and grab your attention. The body survey delivers more, in the long run, for breaking the bonds of reactivity. On the other hand, the benefit of choiceless awareness meditation is that it serves as good training for daily life. Our daily lives contain a composite of one "intrusion" after another—events, emotions, sounds, surprises, joys, and disappointments. Choiceless awareness is thus very useful for its transfer effect to informal practice.

Open Monitoring

Another point on the mindfulness spectrum is what is known as open monitoring. You can practice open monitoring while doing any activity—even simply walking down the street. It is a form of informal practice, in contrast to the formal practices of focused attention and choiceless awareness. With open monitoring, instead of just one object—such as the breath or an emotion—you include *all* these objects in your field of awareness. The difference between choiceless awareness and open monitoring? With open monitoring, *it is the quality of awareness itself that is your anchor.* You are aware of thoughts and feelings arising without establishing any specific point of anchor other than the awareness itself. You abide in awareness—that part of the mind that detects sensations, feeling, and sounds. The aim is to stay in the monitoring state, gently remaining attentive to any experience that might arise.[2]

With open monitoring, you can develop a powerful state of awareness in which you are increasingly present with life's unfolding. You remain open to anything and everything that makes its way through to your conscious awareness, while going about your normal activities. This builds the ability to be fully present with everyday experiences, such as cooking dinner, making the bed, or driving to work.

Practicing open monitoring informally is quite simple. Actually, I am practicing it right now. As I write, I can also hold gentle awareness of the breath, the sensation of my fingers on the keyboard, the morning sun warming my shoulders as it comes through the window, and my body standing or sitting at my desk. The unifying factor is the underlying awareness rather than investigating each phenomenon in depth. Thoughts arise and fall along with sensations in the body and surrounding sounds. With open monitoring, everything as it arises is included in your inventory, without intentionally following any one sensation. Just let it rise and pass.

Open monitoring brings a meditative quality to every action you perform by bringing you into the present. It reduces anxiety and worry, since much of what we worry about isn't actually happening right now. It can be an easy habit to adopt because all it takes is a few meditative moments per day, which soon grow into bringing an element of presence to everything you do.

❧ Mindful Moment: Which Practice, When?

Are you starting to wonder which technique to use when—specific anchor, as with the breath and bodily sensations; choiceless awareness; or open monitoring? The answer is whichever is most appealing, interesting, and best suited to your activity at the time.

Formal practices should be reserved for formal practice time. You don't want to be driving down the freeway while repeatedly returning your full attention to your breath. In such situations, mindfulness means being focused on the task at hand, not being lost in thought or withdrawn from outer engagement, though maintaining awareness of the breath is certainly appropriate. Over time, you will learn which practice best applies when. A little experimentation is welcome and part of the adventure.

Ease and simplicity are paramount. Just because I have provided you with instruction in a few different options for mindfulness practice does not mean you need to do them all to benefit. Far from it.

One type of mindfulness practice is not better or more advanced than another. The best one is that which keeps you present, most skillful in response, and moving toward greater ease. And if sticking with one practice—mindfulness of the breath, for example—works best for you? That's fine, too. If you spend the entire thirty days practicing mindfulness of breath and complete a few body surveys, you are benefitting tremendously and doing wonderfully.

DAY TWENTY-THREE

your naturally healthy body and weight

Perfectionism is not a prerequisite for anything but pain.

—Danna Faulds, poet, yoga teacher, meditator

Meditation Practice: *23 minutes*

Day Twenty-Three, *Meditation on Breath and Bodily Sensations*

Naturally healthy weight. These words bestow such feelings of ease and peace, don't they?

If only we could do that. Find our healthy weight—naturally. What if we could simply sit down to each meal, relish with gusto every delicious bite, set down our forks or chopsticks when our hunger is satisfied, and easily maintain a healthy weight and a happy, harmonious relationship with our body? Without all the angst, struggle, preoccupation, and self-recrimination? Sound like what you are looking for? With mindfulness practice, this can become—as it has for me—your reality. Without the mind-numbing, body-shaming brutality of dieting or focusing on weight loss.

Come to Your Senses

Barring an unusual medical circumstance, you will settle in at your naturally healthy weight when two factors join forces. These factors, your outer and inner senses, are interdependent. They emerge with the increasing conscious connection between mind and body that come with mindfulness.

Outer Sense

Outer sensibility means a basic working knowledge of which foods make it possible for you to naturally satisfy your nutritional needs and hunger, deliver delight in your meals, and inspire your body to be its healthiest. Whole-food, plant-based nutrition accomplishes this best—see The Mindful Vegan Plate (page 116).

Inner Sense

Your inner senses are mindfulness of body, mind, and emotions. Today, we'll look at how hitching up your outer sense (whole-food nutrition) with your inner sense (the feeling of how your body is responding to what and when you eat) is key in realizing your naturally healthy body and weight. Together, your outer and inner sensibilities bring ease and joy into your eating experience. How does the healthy vegan plate meet your innate desire to satisfy your hunger and support your naturally healthy body and weight?

Interoception: A Closer Look

We talked about interoception—your awareness of your body's inner physiological state—on Day Seven, Bodily Sensations. It is your interoception that tells you when you are hungry and when you've had enough to eat. This is accomplished through several mechanisms.

Interoceptors such as the stretch receptors provide a graphic illustration of why whole plant foods are the best match for satisfying your hunger in a way that keeps you at your healthiest. As you eat a whole-food vegan meal—a bean burrito and salad; a bowl of rice and veggie stir-fry; or oatmeal, fruit, and toast with almond butter—it starts making its way through your system. Because these foods are brimming with fiber, they take up space as they progress through your digestive tract, which starts to stretch to accommodate the fiber. When the stretch has reached a certain point, stretch receptors in your gut fire off messages to your brain that say, "Hey, it's getting full down here!"[1] Many of us are in the habit of plowing past this signal, our minds miles away. Yet when you become mindfully attuned to this signal and give it respect, you can then put down your fork, hunger happily satisfied—naturally.

In contrast, highly processed foods, having had the fiber ripped out of them, can hamper this process. And animal products—meats, eggs, and dairy products—have no fiber in them at all. In both cases, due to the stretch factor alone, you can see how it would be easy to eat more than you need before the stretch factor kicks in. Five hundred calories of black beans, rice, and some salad with a chunk of avocado will fill you quite nicely, while it can take more than twice the caloric quantity of fiber-deficient edibles to reach satisfaction. This is why calorie counting and portion control won't work. Unless we meet the body's natural need for the stretch factor, we'll be stuck perpetually trying to eat less than we want. Ever try that before? How'd that work out for you?

Satisfy Nutritional Needs

In addition to the stretch receptors, there are other elements that contribute to hunger satisfaction, and they all command our respect. Your interoceptors are also seeking satisfaction of your nutritional needs—of which fiber is just one part. It also includes sufficient calories, carbohydrate, protein, fat, and an entire array of phytochemicals from plants that are essential for your body to function optimally. It also incorporates awareness of the weight of the food you eat—another job of the gut interoceptors.[2] Let's not forget that your interoceptive sensibilities are also seeking sensory satisfaction from what you eat. That means texture, taste, eye appeal, comfort—all qualities that ask us to be present, mindful, and in a receptive, relaxed state while enjoying each meal.

This is why attempting to use the stretch factor as a way to hack into weight loss, as many diets do, doesn't work. Trying to get by on rabbit food to fool your body into thinking you've had enough will backfire. Without sufficient nutrition—including calories, carbohydrates, proteins, fats, and all the other precious goods that plants deliver—when your hunger overrides your drive to lose an inch off your waist in a hurry, you'll crash. It doesn't deliver full sensory satisfaction and enjoyment of what you eat. Your interoceptors simply won't stand for it. Eventually, your survival instinct will overtake your waning willpower and drive you to the cookie jar. To say nothing of the fact that such tactics have nothing to do with your aspirations to cultivate a healthy, happy relationship with food, eating, and your body.

The Full-Yet-Hungry Scenario

Some people discover that when they start eating a vegan diet and build their plate on primarily minimally processed whole foods, they experience a feeling of being "full," yet they still feel mildly hungry. This can be partly due to the different feeling of fullness that plant foods deliver, without the heaviness or digestive challenges animal products present. Others may experience this after some time, its arising inexplicable. Either way, it's a call to investigate your plate.

If you're just starting out, be mindful of the fact that plant foods are, overall, lower in energy density than processed foods and animal products. This means that you need to eat more of them to meet your nutritional requirements. Our nutritional needs shift and vary over time, and mindfully tuning in is an important foundation of ongoing success.

The full-yet-hungry scenario is unsustainable. Hunger will sooner or later trigger the survival instinct and drive you to go for heaven knows what. This is a call to find out how to bring more satisfaction and balance to your plate. Is your plate full of color and variety with plenty of vegetables and fruits? Are you eating enough of the more energy-dense whole grains or starchy vegetables to meet your energy needs? Are you including enough plant proteins with beans and legumes along with your greens? What about fats? If you have been overzealous in getting them off your plate, you might want to experiment with nudging in higher-fat plant foods such as avocados, olives, nuts, and seeds. Start by adding a little and see if it affects hunger satisfaction. Our nutritional needs can vary over the years, and sometimes what was working for us before isn't cutting it now. One element or another budged up or down in quantity makes all the difference.

Restoring Your Inner Sense

What if you have lost the ability to know when you are really hungry? Or often the bigger problem: you can't quite figure out when you've had enough to eat? What if you find—as I did after years of on-and-off micromanaging my food in one way or another—that you are unable to connect with little else than the feeling of being either starved or stuffed? Is it possible to recover your natural cues and learn when to stop eating in a way that invites your body to discover its naturally healthy weight, while giving you full sensory satisfaction from your meals? When is enough, enough?

People vary on how well they perceive cues to bodily states. If you have been trying to control your diet or your weight with portions, regimented plans, suppressing or ignoring hunger, or constantly trying to "cut back"—punctuated by overeating blowouts—finding fullness may feel elusive. When you have messed with the works for so long by trying to push away or suppress hunger signals, you may be at a loss as to how to trust your body's natural signals to manage your food. Every time we turn the controls over to another diet plan, we unwittingly further distance ourselves from our birthright: eating in harmony with our natural hunger and fullness interoceptors.

You will be happy to know that you can restore a highly functional connection with these signals. Mindfulness practice provides a lifeline to investigating your inner world of feeling, and that includes interoception of fuel signals.[3] It's quite possible that your hunger and fullness interoceptors just need a tune-up.

Fear of Foods and a Mini Meditation

Sometimes, in the process of navigating from hypercontrol of eating to mindful eating, unexpected fears present themselves—fears that may have been running the show from beneath the surface until revealed through mindfulness practice. If eating higher-fat foods, more starchy vegetables, more fruit—you fill in the food blank—or eating to satisfaction brings up fear, anxiety, or some other unsettling emotion, this gives you important information about inner challenges that may be holding you back from true eating freedom. You can address this directly with the mindfulness tools you have been practicing.

Next time you feel fear in connection with eating foods in any category of the mindful vegan plate, it is the perfect time for applying the process of RAIN (page 134). Or, if you notice this conversation here today is bringing up anxieties surrounding food, and you can carve out a few moments, try this mini meditation right now.

Recognition: Become aware of any inner conversation or conflict surrounding a particular food that may have arisen in your mind. Note and acknowledge any tension. Note also any desire to push the uncomfortable feelings away or blame yourself for having them, an urge to distract yourself from them, or a strong desire to eat something. Recognize that a strong emotion is present and no doubt a story that is deeply familiar to you—possibly painfully so. Gently open to what you are experiencing in a kind, nonjudgmental way.

As you tune in to the direct present-moment experience of what is happening in your body and mind via emotions and thoughts, sharpen your focus on the sensations that are arising in your body. How do you know you are feeling fear, anxiety, or a related emotion? What are the qualities of their embodiment? If you have a history of dietary rigidity around the foods in question—mentally putting them off your list in some sort of legalism derived from diets dictating which foods are "allowed" versus "not allowed"—then this response is perfectly understandable. These sensations now become your anchor point for this mini meditation.

Acceptance: With kindness and compassion for yourself, acknowledge whatever is present. Even feeling disheartened or discouraged by the mere presence of these thoughts or feelings—acknowledge that. Acceptance doesn't mean you like the situation or want it to continue. It means you soften and let go of your mental resistance to what is happening. You don't push it away, control it with dietary lockdown (note the urge to do so), or criticize yourself for the push and pull of desire and disdain you may be feeling. This—right here, right now—is ground zero for a problem you may be having around food and eating.

Investigation: Examine the physical sensations that have arisen in your body with the conflict. Note your urge to identify with them—for that is what we have been doing all our lives. With fear as backdrop, you may discover you get pulled into old thinking loops about diet, such as wanting to control food through one authoritarian measure or another. The sensations may show up as a tightening in your throat, a knot in your stomach, or a compelling urge to go to the refrigerator. Stay patiently connected with the experience through the sensations you are feeling in the present.

As you continue investigating the sensations in your emotional center, you may find emotions that you recognize—perhaps shame or sadness that you are a failure or flawed in some way, or that you will never get out of this fear-with-food loop. If this causes you to start thinking through the problem, get out of your head and into your body. Let go and navigate back to the physical sensations. Continue to watch the sensations as anchor point for this mini meditation. Every time your mind wanders back to the thoughts or conflict, or wants to run with the story of an "eating problem"—which you may find hard to resist—kindly bring your attention back to the point of concentration: the sensations in your body that you are feeling in this present moment. If the sensations become too intense, you can shift into breath as anchor for a few moments, and then return.

One of three things will most likely happen. You may find that the sensations of conflict intensify, then wane, then swing back and forth between the two until you are thinking about something else. You may discover an overall lessening of the intensity so that you can get on with your day, stronger in your practice. You may be overwhelmed by ingrained reactivity and just get something to eat. Yet if this is your experience, it is not cause for discouragement. By following the process of this mini meditation, you have created a new response, resulting in nonidentification.

Nonidentification: You have met yourself with more kindness, compassion, patience, and understanding than when on the autopilot of reactivity. You created a little more space between stimulus and reaction—the very space that you are growing and strengthening every day in your formal practice. You start to recognize that this fear you experienced—or whatever other emotional state may have arisen—is a thought, an experience, an emotional state. It is not your set-in-cement truth. It is not who you are.

This mini meditation is a simple, direct process that you can implement any time you feel fear or anxiety bubbling up about foods, fears, or eating, or any other issue for that matter, and in any setting. If your previous reaction has been inner turmoil, getting lost in a story where certain foods are outlaws, or a certainty that you can't control yourself around particular edibles, mindfulness gives you a new option. Being present with the experience in an investigative, curious capacity walks you further into the light of true eating freedom.

꩜ Mindful Moment: Bethany

My friend Bethany, a teacher and vegan cooking instructor, has discovered that her meditation practice is helping her overcome much of her mental struggle and fear with weight, body issues, and food:

> About a year ago I started a meditation practice. While not as consistent as I'd like to be, there have been several long stretches where I was able to meditate daily. What I'm noticing is that I'm not as obsessed over what the scale says and not as obsessed over exercise. I'm trying to stay healthy, eat well, and exercise, but not beat myself up so much over the chocolate go-to or having dessert. I'm becoming more comfortable in my own skin and allow a few extra curves rather than strive to be so lean. I'm trying to not compare my body size to others so much.

Meditation helps me reframe my thought patterns and steer away from negative thinking. One question I ask myself when I start obsessing is, "Is this useful?" Usually not! There's absolutely nothing gained by obsessing or staying stuck in negative thought patterns or ruminations, whether they are centered on body weight or size, "what I ate today," or what is going on in relationships or at work that is creating stress. Meditation is centering and helps me get more in tune with who I am and why I'm here. One result is more peace of mind. Another tends to be more productivity.

There is a lot to be said for letting go of unrealistic or idealistic expectations about what I think my size should or shouldn't be, or whether I allow myself indulgences or not. Still working on balance. That's why, as in yoga, meditation is referred to as a "practice" not intended to be "perfect." I'm gaining better perspective. This is the same body that supported my young motherhood and carried three babies to term, and the same body that supported their nutrition in their early years through nursing. This is the same body that hugged my children close to me when they were little, and provided comfort to them, and holds all of those memories. I wasn't always obsessing over weight or body size during those times; and I was happy with myself and my circumstances!

I still want to be at a healthy weight and to eat well. And I still want to allow myself dessert without beating myself up over it. I'm letting go of some idealistic "perfect" size or weight and learning to embrace the ebb and flow of life more gracefully, including emotional ups and downs, that may or may not call for a piece of chocolate. And I want to be okay with all of it! That's why I will continue with meditation practice and keep working on practicing loving kindness toward myself and my body, as well as toward others.[4]

the pure joy of eating

I meditate because evolution gave me a big brain, but it didn't come with an instruction manual.

—WES NISKER, author and meditation teacher

MEDITATION PRACTICE: *24 minutes*

DAY TWENTY-FOUR, *Meditation on Mindful Eating*

Perhaps no neural hardwiring is as cemented as that associated with the way we eat. Just try changing the speed or altering the style in which you take your meals, and you'll see exactly what I mean. Most of us are accustomed to rarely completing one bite before getting the next mouthful under way. Still chewing bite one, in comes bite two in a sort of layered effect. Or at the least, subsequent bites are hovering on our fork, readying to march into our mouths.

Being truly connected with how hungry and how full your body really is forms the essence of mindful eating. We have the nagging sense that if we could just be present with when we are really hungry and when we are really full, and honor them both, we'd be home free with our health and weight. Yet our habituated eating style and thoughts about eating management undermine our attempts to eat mindfully. You may, for example, have a certain idea about how much you should eat. You may be wedded to portions from a diet from days gone past, afraid of going over or under that amount. This mealtime baggage obscures the connection with your fullness signals and gets in the way of the simple enjoyment of eating.

As a vegan, you have already stepped up to the plate of more conscious eating. Yet how do you bridge the gap between your current eating style and mindful eating? Perhaps the best place to start is to look at the counterpoint to mindful eating: mindless eating.

Mindless Eating

You probably don't need a description of mindless eating. Just for the sake of clarification, are any of the following currently, or have ever been, part of your experience?

- **Eating autopilot:** You sit down for a meal, and though aware that you are eating, before you know it you've cleaned your plate, and you either feel stuffed or have the urge to go find something more to eat. Or both.
- **Transition eating:** You eat as a "transition" activity, such as after arriving home after a busy day, and find yourself gobbling down a stack of cookies before you knew what hit you. Or after dinner, you rapid-fire pound down a dozen dates, overriding fullness.
- **What-the-hell effect:** You eat something "off plan"—whether in quality or quantity—and keep eating because you'd already "messed up."
- **Procrastination plate:** You eat to put off doing something else—consciously or unconsciously.
- **Problem-solver snack:** You eat (or overeat) when you feel upset about something. Or excited about something. Or nervous about something. Or feel bored. Or . . . (fill in the blank).
- **Tech tandemitis:** Habituated to eating while surfing the web, checking your email, or watching TV, you find yourself uncomfortable with *simply eating.*

- **Bare cupboard:** You repeatedly find yourself unprepared with appropriate food to eat—a slip of mindfulness around food that can create difficulties.

Granted, we all eat a bit mindlessly at times—when we're in a hurry or at a social event, for example. The occasional mindless eating episode is not the problem. It's when these moments happen often enough— and continue to haunt us in the form of regret, hampering personal happiness—that it is. Even more, mindless eating has a way of looping in the second-arrow effect in the form of endless after-the-fact self-recrimination.

Before going a step further, to drive home an important point, much of mindless eating is driven by hunger that has been suppressed or ignored. Letting go of undereating and giving up trying to override your natural hunger and fullness signals through restrictive, regimented diets has a distinct impact on mindless eating. Though letting go of these controls takes mindful effort, it is the key to getting out of food jail.

Who's Coming to Dinner?

How often do you dig into a meal and find that your attention is scattered all over the place? You may be preoccupied with multiple tasks (computer, email, phone, social media, texting, analyzing data at work). You might be mulling over the events of the day, or carried away by fantasies or anxieties about the future. These pull you away from the meal that is taking place right in front of you. Add to this the fact that emotions may occur outside of your awareness, and all of a sudden they're driving your eating behavior.[1] These issues are only given mild attention in conventional health and weight-management interventions. Distraction during eating is often mentioned, but we're never given any real tools for changing it. They focus on restriction of caloric intake through one avenue or another, pulling our attention from the real issues.[2]

Eating takes place in the present. Taste is a sensation that takes place in the present. But if you are only peripherally attendant for your meal, you miss more than full enjoyment of what you eat. You miss all the interoceptor satiety signals, create digestive distress, and contribute to health problems. True satisfaction from what you eat includes attention to as well as appreciation and enjoyment of the flavors, textures, and nutrition each eating episode offers.

Mindful Eating

Can't we just learn how to eat in mindful fashion and call it a day? You might wonder why, in a book including mindful eating in its scope, "mindful eating how-to" isn't addressed on the first page. Remember, *eating mindfully is a natural outgrowth of mindfulness practice and mindful living*. Any guide to eating mindfully that starts with tips for the mechanics of mindful eating right out of the gate is missing the boat. Cultivating mindfulness comes first. Then we can understand the eating part.

Checklists abound for the mechanics of how to eat mindfully. They usually include things like chew every bite a certain number of times, avoid overeating, don't skip meals, sit at a table with a nice plate and napkin, blah blah blah.

Look, if we could "not overeat" just by "not overeating," we wouldn't be in this mess. *These outer behaviors will not, by themselves, give you the freedom you are looking for*. Read that last sentence again. This is where these directions about how to eat mindfully—without a more robust understanding of how to leverage mindfulness practice and *actually doing the practice*—only take you so far and fail miserably at creating fundamental change. It just becomes another diet rule that you are trying to obey, and another opportunity to feel bad when you are out of "compliance."

Hunger, Fullness, and an Interoceptive Tune-Up

Mindful eating includes cultivating the ability to recognize and eat when you are hungry, stop when you have eaten enough, and choose foods that are nutritious and enjoyable. Together, they guide you to make decisions about when, what, and how much to eat. Remember our conversation about interoceptive awareness? Sensory receptors get information from within your body, giving you direct information about your moods, emotions, and level of stress. Recall that interoception has a bigger story to tell. Sensory receptors also relay information from your internal organs, including your digestive system. They transmit signals of when you are hungry and when your hunger has been satisfied (recall the stretch receptors), which are keys to realizing your naturally health weight.

As we have been in the habit of eating for every reason under the sun except to satisfy hunger, we've blurred our ability to read hunger signals. Our eating experience has not only gotten all mixed up with an entire arsenal of other triggers to eat, and strong messages not to eat, it has also disconnected us from those signals that tell us it's mealtime or that we've had enough.

With mindfulness you focus on reestablishing your connection with your natural signals. This is a skillful outgrowth of your daily mindfulness practice, particularly from the meditation of bodily sensations. You then implement mindfulness when you eat, as an application of the skills of paying attention. As you recover interoceptive awareness, you open the door to discovering what and how much your body really needs. You dissolve the tension and struggle that are often associated with the eating experience. You enjoy the full pleasure and taste of food and let go of all the judgment around food along with the fear of overeating.

Mindful eating skills are different from the strategies most commonly taught for weight management, such as regimented meal plans, record keeping, and portion control (see Big Diet, Binges, and a Better Way, page 102). In fact, scientists hypothesize that mindless eating explains the poor long-term success of most weight-loss interventions because they focus on the outer behavior tools at the expense of your inner tools.[3]

Across multiple studies, researchers have found a positive relation exists between mindfulness, healthier eating, and weight normalization—even in the absence of specific instruction in mindful eating mechanics. That means the carryover effect from mindfulness practice shows up as respecting and responding to hunger by eating, less impulsive eating, naturally modified consumption, and a preference for healthier foods. You feel more in control of what you eat because eating mindfully takes into account what drives eating habits that are on autopilot, such as eating in reaction to stress and anxiety.[4]

Because of the attention to the sensations in your body, mindfulness practice will, over time, reconnect you with these body signals.

Sometimes you'll get it right; sometimes you won't. Yet if you persist in being attentive, and keep up your practice, the awareness of these body signals will become clearer. You will become more attuned to your hunger and fullness. And sometimes you'll eat just because it's fun, celebratory, or otherwise special. And yes, that's fine, too.

First Step: Eating as Anchor

Before even thinking about shifting anything about your eating style, first, simply observe what takes place at your next meal. Think of it as a meditation on what *is*—just like your meditations on the breath or your bodily sensations. *Don't try to change anything about the manner in which you eat at this next meal.* Simply observe. Are you overhungry or not hungry at all? What is the speed at which you eat? Do you "layer" bites? Do you analyze each plate like a macronutrient science project or calorie competition? Does your food get chewed well? Do you drink down bites with gulps of beverage? Are you tasting your food? Do you like what you are eating? What makes you stop eating—fullness? Or the fact that you run out of food, or reach some pre-measured endpoint?

For the next few meals, simply observe how you eat them in this fashion. Just like your daily meditation practice, this is an opportunity to see things as they are but in the context of mealtime. As you eat, note any other layers that may be present. Are there feelings that color the eating experience? Are you anxious, judgmental, fearful? Be present with whatever arises, noting the tendency to override, push away, judge—even judging judgment! Heavens, what a mess we've made of things.

This simple process of using eating as anchor is your first step into eating more mindfully. As a matter of fact, you are already eating more mindfully because you are being present, with curiosity. This process will teach you a lot about your eating practices. It may be all you need to change your eating experience.

Hunger Signals and STOP

If you would like more guidance, the STOP strategy (page 85) is one way to help link your mindfulness practice with eating. At your next eating experience, use STOP to connect with your hunger signals. With practice, you will be able to do this in seconds.

Stop. Internally, press the pause button.

Take a breath, letting your attention rest on the breath as anchor. This will help you relax and allow you to be more attuned to your hunger interoceptors. You might want to take a couple of deep breaths to help release any present stress.

Next, expand your awareness to include bodily sensations. **Observe** what signals your body may be sending with regards to hunger. Do you have light hunger, or is your stomach growling? Is it hard to detect any hunger? Is that because you aren't really hungry—or have hunger signals become a blind spot for you? If so, another way to discover them is to look at a plate of healthy food and see what your response is. Are you highly interested and want to dive in? Or are you disinterested?

Next, mindfully consider what you want to do with this information. Do you still want to eat? If so, and if you have a choice, what type of food would you like? If you are already about to sit down to a meal, what elements of it most appeal to you? At first, while you are recovering your hunger signals—if indeed your connection with them needs a rewire—this may seem unclear. With practice, you will connect with them.

Proceed. As you sit down to eat, visually take in everything on your plate. Let this moment be an anticipatory celebration. Take in the aromas. Delight in the colors. Anticipate the textures. Relish your good fortune.

As you begin eating, savor every bite. Feel the food on your fork. Notice the burst of flavor as you slowly begin chewing. If you feel tempted to layer the next bite in before you are finished chewing the first, notice that. Can you chew one bite fully and swallow before reaching for the next? This as an opportunity to step out of eating automaticity. Then take the next bite. You can open again and again to seeing the food, feeling the textures, smelling the food, and tasting the flavors.

Notice how the first few bites are especially delicious, particularly if you are very hungry.

Observe any tendency to gobble your food, layering in more mouthfuls before the previous one has had its moment. Perhaps we want to beat everyone else at the table to seconds. But more often rushed eating is due to a few other things. First, you're in a rush anyway as you arrive at your meal and plow into your plate at an accelerated rate. Second, we want that rush of taste, the burst of flavor that comes with the first bite. We somehow think that by shoveling in more food faster we'll get more flavor. Actually, by layering bites we abort the full pleasure of the previous one by running roughshod over it with another forkful. And third, perhaps you have such guilt or shame associated with eating that you want to quickly get rid of the evidence. Slowing down the pace of eating makes you more aware of fullness signals and ultimately gives you greater enjoyment of what you eat. Absorption of food begins in the mouth, and chewing your food well sends satiation signals to the brain—interoception working in your favor. With consistency of practice, you'll get better at mindful eating, and I promise you will enjoy your meals more than ever.

Finding Your Hunger Satisfaction Sweet Spot

If you find that you are having trouble reading fullness signals as you eat, rest assured that with patience and practice you will recover them. It may be that you have fluctuated between feeling starved and stuffed, overriding natural signals more than you think. Once you navigate through the factors that are disconnecting you from your interoception and real enjoyment of food, you will discover that the hunger satisfaction sweet spot is far more pleasureable a place to set down your fork than is being overstuffed. Not because you try to convince yourself of the fact but because this wisdom naturally arises with mindfulness practice. Chronic or compulsive overeating or undereating fall away. And though there will be times that you eat more than you need, either through distraction or by design at a special event, you have taken back the freedom that comes with mindfully managing when you start and stop eating. Not only that, mindfulness skills also allow you to navigate the second-arrow effect—when you find yourself sitting in judgment of "getting it right" or of what or how much you eat. This ability alone was hugely transformative for me.

Reassess your experience of hunger as you continue to eat. Well-known strategies such as "eating to 80 percent full," though wise in theory, aren't much help if you have messed with the works for so long through overeating and undereating, as I had. If all you know is stuffed or starved, where on earth does one begin to look for 80 percent?

Such awareness demands sharp interoception, which comes via mindfulness practice. To assist, I devised an approach grounded in mindfulness that I call finding my hunger satisfaction sweet spot. With consistent mindfulness practice, along with a basic understanding of the brilliant fashion in which whole plant foods meet our hunger satisfaction needs, this approach has allowed me to enjoy my naturally healthy weight range for two decades.

Here's how you know you are approaching your hunger satisfaction sweet spot. It begins with abandoning the suppression or ignoring of hunger signals by eating well regularly. This dissolves the problems associated with what I call "stored" hunger—where you become so ravenous that your animal instincts kick in. Indiscriminate overeating can seize command in the desperate attempt to fuel your brain and body. This is a destructive cycle that will hamper the honing of your fullness signals.

Next, using your sharpening interoceptive skills, become mindful of the changing effect what you are eating has on your body and well-being. As you continue to eat, the food will have lost a little bit of its taste edge. Your hunger will no longer have the urgency it had before you dove into the meal. You will start to feel comfortably content. One way you know you've hit it right is that about an hour after eating, you still feel great. Absent will be feelings of bloat and lethargy or the sense that you had eaten too much. Absent also will be a persisting hunger—the feeling that you didn't have enough, and you need to scavenge for more. No lingering sense of dissatisfaction, accompanied by repeated return visits to the kitchen, as you find yourself opening the fridge grazing for just the right bite to make that meal feel complete. Just like the story of Goldilocks and the Three Bears, you'll know you hadn't eaten too much, nor too little. Your interoception system will tell you that you ate "just right." Your body told you when you had had enough—which it always does; you just don't always hear or listen to it—and this time you listened. And if it's something else that is driving an interest in more food—stress or another disquieting state—your mindfulness practice gives you the tools for skillfully steering your way through.

As you get better at reading the signals your body sends, you discover your hunger satisfaction sweet spot. Sometimes you, like me, will get it just right, though, like me, not every time. But I've gotten it right often enough to keep a sizeable weight loss from rebounding after nearly twenty years.

If a big gap currently exists between you and your fuel signals, either hunger or fullness, now is the time to cultivate kindness for yourself. Bring the same attitude of patience and compassion to your eating experience that you bring to your meditations. If you don't get it right the first time—which I certainly didn't—it doesn't matter because you can enjoy the adventure to the sweet spot the next time you eat. With your next meal, observe as you are eating when you reach what you think might be a match for the sweet spot. That place where you know that even in an hour, you will feel wonderfully satisfied. Not too full. Not still hungry. Just right. Keep a relaxed and open attitude about the investigation. See it as a discovery process. And when it feels right, even if there is still food on your plate, gently put down your eating utensil.

With the mindfulness that you are practicing every day, this experience will become your new eating norm rather than the exception. When we eat absentmindedly, or are distracted from enjoying our meal by entertainment or rigid controls and judgments about what we are eating, the sweet spot is elusive. We're not really fulfilled by our meal because we're not really there for it. Mindful eating starts as you become more practiced at being present, paying attention to actual experience. Developing the skills of noting tendencies of thought, feeling, and bodily sensation gives you the tools you need to implement these same tools for freedom at the table. Your increasing awareness of and response to your internal cues explains how mindfulness leads to better food choices, happier meals, and your naturally healthy body.

🪷 Mindful Moment: Embodying New Eating Behaviors

As you start investigating your connection with your hunger and fullness signals, you will no doubt encounter a variety of inner responses. You may experience excitement and happiness at letting go of the massive burden of mental controls you've layered onto your meals. Yet don't be surprised if there is also some mental discomfort when you aspire to follow your inner directives. Each of these responses delivers sensations that can be anchor points for mindful attention.

If you are used to eating fast, slowing down might seem tough and a bit awkward. After all, it's not what you are used to. The best way to navigate this discomfort is to use it as a point of observation, just like any other sensation you might anchor with during meditation. What feelings are you having that you associate with taking the rush out of mealtime? Do you feel hampered or constricted? How do you know? How does that show up? Instead of avoiding or burying the discomfort, be fully aware of it, and explore it with curiosity. It is just as any other thought or sensation. Acceptance, investigation, and a willingness to be present with the uneasiness of the changing norm leads to freedom.

Letting go of dietary regimentation can be scary business. After all, you are doing something new, which means you are stepping outside of your comfort zone. This is the perfect opportunity for mindfulness. Bring your attention to any discomfort you are feeling in your body that arises from changing your previous pattern. Perhaps you are used to plowing through to the end, when your plate is empty. Or you may feel discomfort because you are stepping outside the "rules" of portion control. To be honest, this is what propelled me with the most earnestness into practicing mindfulness. I had decided I couldn't do "dieting" anymore. I could not have made the change without these essential key players: whole-food plant nutrition and mindfulness practice.

DAY TWENTY-FIVE

cravings

*The faculty of voluntarily bringing back a wandering attention,
over and over again, is the very root of judgment, character,
and will. No one is compos sui—master of oneself—if he has it
not. An education which should improve this faculty would be
the education par excellence.*

—WILLIAM JAMES

MEDITATION PRACTICE: *25 minutes*

◁)) DAY TWENTY-FIVE, *Meditation on Breath and Bodily Sensations*

 Ever reach for edible comfort when stressed? Certain you are addicted to food? For the next couple of days, we'll look at cravings, related concerns about addiction, and why traditional control-based strategies to deal with them haven't been more successful. You'll find out how a focus on restrictive eating may have been working against you, and what the research says about the success of a mindful approach to all of it.

Consider the following scenarios:

SCENARIO A: Breakfast is only halfway eaten when a quick glance at the clock tells you you'd better get a move on. It seems there's never enough time to do all you want to before heading out the door in the morning. Quickly, you toss your dishes in the sink. In your haste your favorite mug slips from your hand, fatally chipping the drinking rim. Dang. You pick up the fragments and flip on the garbage disposal to empty the food scraps in the sink, only to find that the disposal hums but doesn't want to get to work and grind. Oh great, you think. Another home maintenance issue.

Agitated, you finish getting dressed, grab your keys, and check the time, realizing you are probably going to be late for your appointment. Turning on the car ignition, you notice the gas gauge light is on. You realize that, because you now have to stop for gas, you'll be late for sure. As you pull out of the driveway, suddenly—from out of what seems like nowhere—visions of your favorite pastry and hot drink pop into your mind. You can smell it, taste it. Oh, would that be good, you think. The bakery is right on the way. Maybe you can dash in and grab it before your appointment.

Then the familiar inner arguments start. You've been doing so well with your food the last three days, you tell yourself. You don't really want to blow it with a mini splurge, yet how much can one pastry hurt? You didn't get to finish breakfast anyway, you ruminate, but what if this indulgence sets you off for a few days because you are, after all, so addicted to sweets? You try to fan the flames of motivation for your healthy change plan that was so strong yesterday. But the embers have burned out, and you can't get it rekindled for the life of you. Now engaged in full-on combat with a craving for that midmorning treat (that you so well deserve after all you've been through this morning!), yet knowing that it is not in line with your best-laid plans and resisting giving in with all your might, you...

SCENARIO B: Breakfast is only halfway eaten when a quick glance at the clock tells you you'd better get a move on. It seems there's never enough time to do all you want to before heading out the door in the morning. Quickly, you drop the rest of your nut-buttered toast into a bag to enjoy on the drive. As you hastily toss your dishes in the sink, your favorite mug slips from your hand, fatally chipping the drinking rim. Dang. You immediately note the disappointment in your mind and the tightness you feel in your stomach in reaction. Staying present with these sensations, you pick up the mug fragments and flip on the garbage disposal to empty the food scraps in the sink, only to find that the disposal hums but doesn't want to get to work and grind. Oh great, you think, another home maintenance issue. Before inner drama even has a chance to get started, you implement STOP (page 85). You pause, take a breath, and observe the sensations in your body that alert you to stress. You note the interest your mind has in running with the "It's going to be one of those days!" story lines. Keeping mindful of the unsettling race of thoughts that have been arising in your mind and the accompanying reactions in your body, you stay connected with the calm beneath the surface storm as you proceed. While acknowledging agitation is present, you are not engulfed in its jaws.

Proceeding, you finish getting dressed, grab your keys and breakfast leftovers, and check the time—aware of the fact that you are probably going to be late for your appointment. Switching on the car ignition, you notice the gas gauge light is on. You now realize that since you have to stop for gas, you'll be late for sure. As you pull out of the driveway, suddenly—from out of what seems like nowhere—visions of your favorite pastry and hot drink pop into your mind. You observe and intercept this development. Turning your awareness to your thoughts and urge for quick comfort, you simultaneously attend to the sensations in your body that are communicating stress, emotional reactivity, and desire. While observing these phenomena as they are arising, and being present with them, you arrive at the gas station. Your thoughts have turned to realizing it would probably be a good idea to call and tell your appointment that you are running a bit late. You notice that the craving for the comfort stop at the bakery is less urgent, having lost its compelling nature. You become aware of hunger, signaling you to turn to your unfinished breakfast—the toast and nut butter—which you start eating as you pull out of the station.

While the specifics may be different from your exact experience—I pulled the particulars of this scenario from my own—perhaps you recognize this familiar unfolding of a food craving just the same. Which is more familiar to you: Scenario A? Or is scenario B more like your experience? What's the difference between the two?

Scenario A depicts careening through stress with reactivity. Stress accumulates with reactivity to one mini incident after another, pinball-style, building with no relief until you reach your breaking point. In contrast, scenario B demonstrates mindful intervention. This is achieved by applying skills of mindful awareness—the same skills that you have been practicing every day. Rather than getting caught up in every mini event, you observe the unfolding of circumstances while staying aware of the mental, emotional, and physical processes arising in the midst of these incidents. This gives you fraction-of-a-second opportunities for a fresh response to stress as you go. Being willing to be present, you note the choices. You can go with reactivity. Or you can be mindfully present throughout the unsettling series of episodes—completely different from telling yourself you should calm down or that you shouldn't feel a certain way. Do you see how overcoming the habits of reactivity in this way might lead to living with greater ease, happier outcomes, and more skillful living?

Of course, we'd all rather have rush-free mornings and long, luxurious breakfasts. But they aren't always the default, and we can find ourselves in a situation similar to the scenarios described above more often than we like. Your response, however, can be shifted with mindfulness practice. You can create responses more along the lines of scenario B, giving you better outcomes to a rushed morning.

When your new response, as a result of regular mindfulness practice, is the willingness to be present with whatever is taking place and to navigate the discomfort, it gets even better. It can eventually lead to scenario C—where the idea of the pastry as you pull out of the drive doesn't even materialize. The thought, if it does come up, will be intercepted earlier, in the form of a rising energy, before it fully takes form. Or it will simply not bubble up at all as you become mindfully present at an earlier point in the unfolding scene. This doesn't mean you never feel uneasy. It means you have tools to navigate stress more skillfully. Does this sound like the kind of freedom you'd like to experience?

Cravings Ground Zero

Understanding where cravings come from sheds light on why mindfulness makes the difference between being commandeered by cravings versus being able to intercept and manage their arising skillfully. Mindful eating includes learning to detect and honor hunger signals. As you get better at this, being blindsided by what we might call a craving but is actually real hunger will naturally subside. Not to be confused with a strong drive to eat caused by hunger, cravings are characterized by an intense yearning for specific foods or other substances, whether or not accompanied by hunger. Once you have insight into the origins of cravings—and tools for getting out of the painful jam they put you in—the shackles of food cravings loosen and fall away.

Cravings—or what we perceive as cravings—can be generated by deprivation, environmental cues, and emotional reactivity. Let's take a look at all three and the mindfulness response. Mindfulness has proven to be an effective antidote for all of them.[1]

Deprivation

According to the research, being deprived of foods you enjoy can lead to cravings. As soon as you swear off chocolate, you want it more than ever! Losing variety in your daily menu can contribute to the sense of deprivation, too. Both self-restriction and monotony are associated with increased food craving experiences.[2] If you are new to becoming vegan, this may also include old omnivore favorites that have been highly rewarding to the pleasure centers of your brain.

Several strategies serve as antidote to cravings that arise from deprivation. Preventatively, pay attention to eating vegan foods and flavors that you like. Eating mindfully, you can enjoy what is called sensory-specific satiety. This means you can maximize enjoyment of your favorite foods in what often turns out to be moderate quantities. You pay attention to satisfying hunger with the flavors you love—absent the layers of judgment, fear, and angst that separate you from reading fullness signals and true satisfaction. If there are dishes from your pre-vegan days that you really liked and miss, there are lots of resources on the internet and in cookbooks that show you how to re-create those same flavors and textures with vegan ingredients. Some people create strict rules around whether they can have even a bite of specific foods, even though they are vegan. Some can tolerate this approach or find it helpful. For others it reinforces problematic black-or-white thinking. Dietary rigidity can amplify dietary disinhibition—a letting go of and defiance of all controls.[3] This is why white-knuckle, "just say no" strategies can be so hit or miss.

In short, if you are pounding down a quart of collard greens because you know they are good for you, but you can't stand the taste, find another way to get the nutrition that you are eating the greens for. Give up eating punitively. Be kind and nurturing to yourself by eating delicious, nonmonotonous meals. Create more variety in what you eat, with both flavor and texture. Remember that eating mindfully makes it possible for you to enjoy your favorite vegan meals and treats, too, should you so choose. Should feelings of deprivation persist, implement RAIN to navigate how they are showing up as thoughts and feelings.

External Food Cues

The sight or smell of food—even the mere thought of eating—can be enough to start your body gearing up for a meal. It is your body's way of getting primed to better absorb and use the nutrients that might soon be on the way.[4] From an evolutionary perspective, this makes sense. After all, if your ancestors weren't tuned in to the food availability in the

206 • the mindful vegan

environment, they might just pass it by and miss a rare opportunity to refuel. While some people interpret this response as a craving, it's simply a normal reaction to the fact that edibles are at hand, giving reason for the desire to eat that may accompany it.[5]

Simply being mindful of the "food cue" phenomenon helps you skillfully navigate it. Observe the peaked interest in eating that is taking place, take note of how it affects your thoughts, and investigate your physical response in bodily sensations. Check to see if you are simply hungry. Note if you have the impulse to upgrade this natural interest in eating to urgent status by calling it a "crave." You can then pick skillfully from your options. You can decide, mindfully, to eat something. Or if hunger isn't the issue, you can watch the urge to eat rise and fall away, rather than creating more tension and giving it more strength by trying to push it away or resist it. This is quite different from "just say no" and trying to bury the rising desire or talk yourself out of feeling a certain way. With mindfulness you bring your attention to the experience and navigate it with conscious awareness. The effect is changed pathways in the brain as you morph from reactivity to wise response.

Emotional Reactivity

Food cravings are highly correlated with eating in response to emotions and are closely associated with mood. Dysphoric moods such as restlessness, depression, and even boredom precede the cravings themselves—think complications of the default mode network—and cravers can experience higher ratings of anxiety.[6]

Due to past practices, we are being urged, via craving, to distract ourselves from or relieve the stress-induced discomfort by seeking reward or relaxation. This response to negative emotions ("I'm sad and I want something to eat!"—often a player in binge eating) can give rise to cravings ("I'm upset and need chocolate NOW!"—the stress-hedonic eating model).[7] Cravings for certain edibles such as processed sweets, salty snacks, and cheese can arise because eating them triggers the release of a heightened pleasure cycle—via the brain's biochemical reward system—that quells anxiety, subdues anger, soothes stress, and even generates feelings of euphoria. That's why we usually crave chocolate more than we do Brussels sprouts. To make things worse, this entire food-as-reward-system that is wired to your brain biochemistry is driven by habits.[8] Let's say the memory of a particular edible—chips, cookies, or ice cream—comes to mind. It has rescued you from pain in the past, so it's a safe bet it can do the same thing again. So when it's three o'clock, you're stressed, and visions of the new Ben and Jerry's vegan ice cream flavor dance into your mind, it's probably because that's what you've indulged in at the three o'clock stress point before. Habit-driven comfort. Without an antidote, against our better judgment, and overlooking or temporarily blinded to the misery that follows, we cave.[9]

Managing food cravings so that they do not lead to even more emotional distress or unhealthy food consumption is critical to finding peace with food. Craving is an *affective* state.[10] That means it can be mindfully regulated just as any affective state. An affective state is one in which your feelings control your consciousness. When a craving—remember, we're not talking about real hunger and a genuine need for food here—strikes from what seems like out of the blue, your frame of mind is being commandeered by your feelings—deprivation, desire, anxiety, or any other emotions that may have arisen. Before you know it, cravings surface. They intrude your thoughts with annoying strength and persistence, often in the form of cravings for specific, rich foods. We all know the feeling.

We typically react to cravings in one of three ways:

1. Indulge in the craving. This brings immediate excitement and relief, yet it also brings along a lot of baggage in the form of misery—pain follows right on the heels of the fun. It also reinforces the craving habit loop.
2. Distract ourselves. This may take the form of eating something healthier instead (known as surrogacy, often followed by eating the original craved food later anyway), surfing TV or the internet, or trying to talk ourselves out of it by stirring up shame in one of its many guises.
3. Dig in our heels to resist it. As I recently heard a health coach tell his following, "Gut it out." How does one do that, anyway? Gut it out? Where are the instructions?

How to Control Cravings by Simply Paying Attention

Why bury the bomb when you can disarm it? In study after study, mindfulness-based interventions have been shown to have dramatic positive effects on cravings.[11] The biggest benefit of simply observing with mindful attention, as you are doing with formal mindfulness practice, is that you interrupt mindless impulses that can show up as stress-eating habit loops. You are modulating the link between stimulation and reaction, opening up the space between them, presenting the opportunity to make another choice.[12]

How exactly does mindfulness help you step out of this habit loop? First, during mindfulness practice, you are learning to observe your thoughts as transient events. As you pay close attention to cravings, you start to see that they are actually an amalgamation of bodily sensations and thoughts. You begin to notice these phenomena as they appear, and how they can morph from moment to moment. Just as with any other thought or sensation, you discover you can let them go, watch them defuse, or ride their course observantly, rather than try to squash them or get carried away by them. Being observable, it's workable.

As cravings arise, pay attention to how they are showing up. The increased awareness of bodily sensations and emotions as you have started to practice is essential here. The most direct line to navigating cravings skillfully is to discover where and how you are feeling them in your body. Implement RAIN. *Recognize* that craving is arising or has surfaced. *Acknowledge* and *accept* that craving is present. Remember, acceptance is not indulgence. It is necessary for making change. *Investigate* the signs of craving and how craving shows up in your body as physical sensations. If you can't connect with the sensations right away, the body survey is made for this moment. You can do a quick scan in a matter of seconds. Gather your attention at the top of your head, and go. Note the information your body is giving you about your current state. Rather than "gutting it out," you investigate craving mindfully by dropping beneath the surface turbulence and looking craving straight in the eye where it manifests in thoughts, emotions, and sensations, steadfastly staying aware of how the turmoil is playing itself out.

As you stay fully present with the physical experience of what craving feels like in your body, one or more of several things will happen. You will become aware of the physical sensations that you didn't even notice a moment ago. You may discover that your thoughts keep pulling you back to what it is you are craving. Acknowledge that, and kindly get right back into your body. It may feel very uncomfortable, as if you are in the middle of a battle zone. Instead of the old method of trying to win the skirmish via willpower, be present with the conflict—walking right through the middle of it. You'll come out fine. Trust me. You will start to realize that not only will craving not last forever, but it is simply a bundle of thoughts and feelings. Through this process, *nonidentification* with the craving takes place. You may find that in a few moments your mind has left the battlefield and is already planning dinner. This shows you the ephemeral nature of things like cravings.

In the beginning, you may find that, minutes later, you are still experiencing mental and physical conflict. You may even stay present with it all for a few minutes and then cave to the crave anyway. Even if this happens, you have set a precedent of awareness. You have started a new in-the-moment practice. You have underscored and realized the importance of those precious minutes of formal mindfulness practice that prepare you like nothing else can for this very moment. Be present with whatever it is you are eating and enjoy it! You may note that this is a time when the second-arrow effect loops in. Another opportunity for being mindfully present.

With practice, and staying consistent with your meditation, this will become your new operating mode. You will be able to observe the playing out of the sensations of craving in your body. At some point your mindful presence will have become practiced enough so that you will be aware of sensations building up even before cravings crash to the surface. Not every time, but with more and more consistency, relative to practice. Other than your daily formal practice, this is the single most powerful tool in your mindfulness toolkit for getting through difficulties: drop your attention right into your body and navigate the moment. In this fashion, you are acknowledging everything about your condition, which downregulates inner conflict and positions you for making more skillful choices.

Mindfulness sharpens your powers of observation so you can be on the lookout for the ways in which you might be feeding these habits and craving loops. Each time you become mindful of a craving and step out of the loop—a simple attention shift—it gets weaker. Learning to manage your attention is one of the most potent aspects of meditation practice. It is indispensable to learning how to respond to cravings in a fresh way.

The frequency of being at the mercy of cravings will lessen until they become, more and more often, a scenario B. And eventually a scenario C. Your body can teach you so much. It is a trustworthy guide. Eventually, via mindfulness, cravings diminish and then disappear. They dim like the harbor fading into the distance as your vessel pulls out to sea. And you have lifelong tools for working with them should they arise at some other point in your life. Mindfulness disarms the war with food and your body and restores the pure joy of eating, letting you out of eating prison and giving you the kind of freedom of experience you are looking for.

Samantha, a legal assistant and one of my students, shared her experience of the effects of working mindfully with cravings:

> I had been plagued by a craving for ice cream every night after dinner since my mom died two years ago. The connection was obvious. It was a family tradition to enjoy a bowl of ice cream every evening. Even though I knew where my nightly craving was coming from, I didn't know what to do to stop it. I would try to resist the craving and that would last for a couple of days, maximum. I knew about the properties of dairy products that made ice cream more compelling to eat, too.
>
> I had been practicing mindfulness meditation for about two weeks when I found my way out of this problem. I was having lunch with a friend who asked me how I was doing with regards to my mom. I told her that it was still really hard, and that "the pain is almost palpable."
>
> As soon as I heard the words come out of my mouth it was like a light bulb went off. I had just started learning meditation of bodily sensations. So as the feelings came up, I turned my attention directly to what it felt like, palpably, to miss my mom so much. My stomach was knotted and my throat got instantly tight.

We continued our lunch and I put the information away for later to explore the next time I got the craving for ice cream. Sure enough, when the craving came up, I turned my attention to what it felt like in my body. The first day I ate ice cream anyway. By the third day, watching the sensations in my body when the craving arose and being present with the pain of grief for my mother, I started to see the pull to the ice cream for what it was and that there might just be the possibility of choice in the matter. For a few days after that, I was aware of the memory of the craving and would watch the sensations. After a week, when the idea of ice cream came up in the evening, I could see it as simply a thought and go directly to where it had created a craving response in my body. Soon, the craving was completely unraveled. Now, I occasionally enjoy vegan ice cream—but without all the painful connections, impulsivity, and the problems that dairy presents. I still miss my mom, but now it is not compounded by the pain of eating something I regret. No wonder they call this "insight" meditation.[13]

❁ Mindful Minute: Mindful Attention Quickly Prevents Mindless Eating Impulses

As much as I want you to understand how daily dedicated practice to mindfulness will give you the most far-reaching benefits for managing reactivity, mindfulness can be leveraged to prevent mindless eating impulses right out of the gate. Three studies illustrate that mindful attention can prevent impulses toward compelling food, even with no prior practice.

Participants received brief mindfulness instructions just moments prior to the experiment. They were directed to observe their reactions to external stimuli as transient mental events, rather than subjectively real experiences—the same as you are practicing every day in meditation. Specifically, when presented with appealing foods, they were instructed to watch their internal reaction as a phenomenon, without identifying with their reactions. Across all experiments, reactions were fully eliminated for subjects in the mindful attention group compared to the control group, who did not receive the instructions on modulating attention mindfully. Researchers concluded that mindful attention to our own mental experiences *as simply mental experiences* helps to control impulsive responses, demonstrating mindfulness as a powerful method for self-regulation even if you are new to practice.[14] How's that for an encouraging word?

DAY TWENTY-SIX

addiction, part one

*The interesting thing is that we all carry this peace within.
Everyone has it. Yet there are constant wars going on
in ourselves, our families, in the workplace...between
nations. But all the time this peace rests within us. We need
only concentrate to find it...Experiencing our own inner
peacefulness and learning to return to it again and again is
enough to change the entire quality of our lives.*

—Ayya Khema, *Who Is My Self*

Meditation Practice: *26 minutes*

Day Twenty-Six, *Meditation on Breath and Bodily Sensations*

While the research surrounding mindfulness as an antidote to cravings is consistently positive, what about addictions? If we can modify cravings with mindfulness, shouldn't it follow that it would also have the potential to affect addictions?

The answer is yes. The research surrounding the positive effect of mindfulness training on binge eating disorders, substance use disorders, depression, and other medical conditions has shown such promise that scientists are studying its role in treating addictions. Today we'll look at recent research about the effect of mindfulness training on the granddaddy addiction of them all—smoking—and how it outperformed the American Lung Association's program for smoking cessation. You'll find out how the mechanisms of mindfulness—and the effect they have on cravings, a core element to addiction of any kind—were key.

Whether or not smoking is or has been an issue for you, the example of mindfulness practice for dealing with smoking addiction is highly illuminating for other forms of substance challenges, including food, which is why the exciting research is presented in such detail here. An inability to suppress a behavior, despite the behavior's negative consequences, is common in addiction. Suppress is a key word to note here, as you will see with this example of mindfulness training for smoking addiction, for nonsuppression is one of the qualities of mindfulness.[1-2]

Mindfulness Training and Addiction

In this smoking-cessation study, eighty-eight treatment-seeking subjects who were smoking an average of half a pack of cigarettes a day were randomly assigned to either Freedom From Smoking, a standard quit-smoking program, or mindfulness training.[3] Standard smoking-cessation programs typically use a behavioral approach. They focus on strategies such as avoiding smoking triggers (don't have cigarettes in the house or hang out with other smokers or go where you might encounter the possibility of having a cigarette); diverting attention from cravings by distracting yourself with other activities; substituting other items for smoking (chewing on a carrot); reducing stress; and getting social support. If you see the similarity between this list of tactics and the behavioral approach reviewed in Day Twelve: Big Diet, Binges, and a Better Way (page 102), it is because it is based on the same model. Just as in weight-loss programs, these stop-smoking programs have shown only modest success, with abstinence rates hovering between 20 and 30 percent. It's pretty much all we've had to go on. Until now.

The mindfulness training group in this study practiced formal mindfulness meditation at home for about twenty minutes a day on the average of five days a week. Through meditation on the feeling of the breath and bodily sensations, they learned how cravings feel in the body and how mindfulness training can help you become more aware of these processes as they arise. They observed how thoughts, emotions, and body sensations become triggers for craving and smoking, and learned the RAIN technique to mindfully approach cravings. They discovered in what ways difficult emotions perpetuate smoking and learned to practice loving-kindness meditation (page 163) as a way to work with them. They also went about their daily activities mindfully as much as possible.

To level the playing field, treatment for both groups were matched in duration and follow-up. All training sessions were delivered by instructors experienced in either Freedom From Smoking program protocol or mindfulness training, respectively. Everyone was given a training manual and home practice materials, which were matched for amount of audio support.

Mindfulness Training Twice as Effective

Mindfulness training proved to be *twice as effective* as the behavioral approach in helping people treat smoking addiction. A significant reduction in cigarette use resulted during treatment and was maintained through the seventeen-week follow-up.

The game changer? The smokers in the mindfulness training group were taught how to pay attention to, and be present with, their cravings. They learned that cravings are, when you get right down to it, made up of bodily sensations: tension, restlessness, and agitation. They learned that these sensations, which had been driving their lives, come and go. They learned how to be aware of cravings as they arise and then go away, and that they didn't have to get pulled in by them *or* resist them.

Mindfulness Training and the Addictive Loop

Taking a play-by-play look at the flow of reactivity, known as the addictive loop, in smoking addiction, you can see the fundamental difference between the standard treatment and the mindfulness training approaches:

The Addictive Loop

1. Stimulus to smoke: positive (good meal), negative (boss yells at you), or neutral (you get in your car, a time when you usually light up a smoke)
2. Urge to smoke
3. Craving for cigarette
4. Smoking, thus reinforcing the loop

Standard treatments such as the Freedom From Smoking program seek to intervene first by avoiding stage one, situations that previously triggered smoking cravings. Should that fail, the next intervention is between steps three and four, craving and smoking, via substitute behaviors (e.g., chewing gum).

There are two problems inherent with this approach that explain the high failure rate. First, avoiding stimulus that might inspire the urge to smoke. Avoid good meals, arguments, settings, and all other circumstances to which you have hardwired smoking? How do you do that? Second, once craving has kicked in, you substitute some other behavior to try to satisfy the urge to smoke. In this case, you have not addressed the fundamental problem—craving. You are still bound by reactivity; you just found something to substitute for the original offender. This reinforces the craving cycle. For most, it's only a matter of time before the old substance sneaks its way in. You can still avoid situations that inspire you to smoke, though that might be impossible to fully achieve.

With mindfulness training, the intervention emphasis happens at the point when craving arises in a way that dissolves the craving itself. It disassembles the craving flow, putting an end to the cycle rather than perpetuating it with a substitute or locking oneself away to avoid any possible cravings arousal. Through mindfulness training, the smokers learned to be present with negative sensations, cravings, and withdrawal—without reacting to these unpleasant states as was their habit: smoking. Mindfulness training cultivated their ability to recognize these as transient feelings and sensations in the mind and body—rather than something that is happening to them—and label them as craving. They learn not to identify with everything surrounding the event but to be able to work with it as an experience—an extension of thoughts as objects. Remember: if it's observable, it's workable. The mindfulness training dampened and eventually dismantled the complex interrelated processes of smoking rather than just removing circumstances that contribute to the urge.[4]

This same approach applies to food. Instead of trying to eat carrots instead of cookies or avoiding going anywhere near "trigger" foods, through mindfulness you skillfully navigate the entire flow, dissolving the "addicted to food" cascade.

Over the past century, much has been discovered about the addictive process and its underlying neurobiology.[5] Neuroimaging tells us that basic processes, such as default-mode-network activation patterns, can be altered in a fundamental way with mindfulness training through changing one's relationship to core addictive elements such as craving. The shift from "reacting" to the "skillful responding" of mindfulness—a result of observing, nonjudgment, and nonreactivity—decreases craving and a need to alleviate its discomfort with substance use. It increases acting with awareness and intentional behavior.[6]

During mindfulness practice, you monitor unskillful thought processes and automatic behaviors. You learn to observe behaviors—such as smoking or engaging in unhealthy eating—objectively, rather than be "sucked in" by them. The more you are able to uncouple craving from behavior through mindfulness practices, the less they foster the addictive loop. This leads to the cessation of craving itself.

The very same things neuroscientists are discovering about our brains, and how we can disassemble problematic habits, parallel what mindfulness practice brings to the table.[7] In mindfulness terms, that means: 1) self-regulation of attention and 2) orientation to the experience—specifically maintaining an attitude of acceptance toward the experience. This targets the addiction loop in two ways. It brings habits into consciousness so that you can work with them, and it targets the learning process with an emphasis on effect and craving as critical components of positive and negative reinforcement loops.[8]

When we start to see really clearly what happens when we get caught up in our habits of thinking, they loosen their grip. As we become willing to be present with our experience, rather than pushing away the unpleasant (like cravings), acting on it, or distracting ourselves from it, old habits fall away as we form a new practice of being mindfully present. We step out of the process of reactivity by being attendant and curiously aware of what's happening, quieting down the craving region of the brain.

Mindful Moment: Breaking a Bad Habit Mindfully

I had developed a habit of cruising the bulk bins at a local natural foods store whenever I went there to shop. I had a particular penchant for the dark chocolate covered almonds. It got so that every time I went to this store, I found myself clutching a bag of them, whether I was hungry or not. I literally could no longer shop at this store without getting and eating a bag of them. I told myself I was addicted to chocolate. As often as I had said to myself I would "not do that this time," I would be drawn to the bin nonetheless. I considered that perhaps I should not shop there anymore.

Mindfulness practice changed this for me. I decided that the next time I went to this store I would practice what I had started to do in meditation. As I approached the store, I could see, for the first time, the desire and craving for the chocolate almonds arising in my mind, and the cravings start. Instead of identifying with the craving as I did before, I realized I could see it as a phenomenon, and I opened my awareness to what was going on in my body. I could see the whole thing unfolding—the physical desire, in anticipation of the rewards of the chocolate. I could feel the strong pull to follow through and go grab a bag of the nuts. Rather than try to fight it, which had never worked in the past, I decided to stay with observing the physical response I was having to the idea of eating the chocolate almonds. Every time my mind went back to the thought of getting them, I turned my attention back into the physical experience of the craving. This had the dramatic effect of loosening the grip this obsession had on my mind and body. The closer I looked, the more I was present with the experience—rather than being caught up in the fight that can accompany "guilty pleasure"—the more relaxed I felt as it started to soften its hold on my attention. Then I noticed I had forgotten about it! This brought it back to mind, so I simply approached it in the same way again. Accepting, watching, investigating. I could notice the latent desire, but I also noticed I had a new freedom of choice. I could see how it was possible to be at ease with not getting a bag of the mix. I continued to attend to this process off and on through this particular trip to the store. And lo and behold, I didn't buy a bag! Something had shifted, and it wasn't just talking myself out of getting a treat.

The next time I went to this store, I went through the same process. But the strength of the pull to past habits had weakened and it was easier than the first time. I now have a much better idea of what "acceptance" with mindfulness really means. It has nothing to do with giving in to indulgences! It has to do with giving up a fight that I could never win by approaching inner conflict in a whole new compassionate, mindful way.

—RICHARD SULLIVAN, DVM

DAY TWENTY-SEVEN

addiction, part two

*Rather than converting people from one organized religion to
another organized religion, we should try to convert people
from misery to happiness, from bondage to liberation,
and from cruelty to compassion.*

—S. N. GOENKA

 MEDITATION PRACTICE: *27 minutes*

🔊 DAY TWENTY-SEVEN, *Meditation on Breath and Bodily Sensations*

People who are haunted by food cravings often feel with a certainty that they are addicted to food. Addictions are, as we know, characterized by cravings. Scientists are still debating whether food or obesity qualify as addictions. There is a lot of dissention about how to define them, what foods might qualify as addictive, and how to tease them apart from other lifestyle factors that may play a role. As evidence for addiction to specific macronutrients in humans is lacking, scientists suggest the term *eating addiction* might be more appropriate, as it describes a behavioral addiction.[1]

Today we'll explore the phenomenon popularly known as food addiction and the comparison of control-based (standard behavioral) and acceptance-based (mindful) strategies to address it.

The Outliers

First, let's take some of the outliers off the table. There are studies suggesting specific biochemically driven reasons for why some people feel out of control with eating. Self-assessed food addicts who say they suffer from "volume addiction" or "overeating of all foods" may have low leptin levels that contribute to a strong urge to eat and binge on everything. Or they may have an insulin disorder. People with celiac disease can experience lack of hunger satisfaction for completely different biochemical reasons. Clinically, these situations are the rare exception rather than the rule.[2]

Food "Addiction" Cofactors

Some binge eaters experience cravings for foods suspected as being most "addictive": sugar, fat, refined flour, salt, and artificial sweeteners. We know that foods rich in fat and sugar can supercharge the brain's reward system, toying with our interest in telling ourselves to stop eating as levels of dopamine and its cohorts in our feel-good biochemistry rise. These responses that are linked with food reward can play a role in excessive food consumption.

Yet taking these observations from the lab at face value is short-sighted. It begs the question: What is the diet history of the subjects? Most people who feel that they are food addicts often have complicated diet histories. Periods of restrained eating, off and on dieting (in some instances, for years—guilty!), or some other variation of disturbed or disordered eating may be part of the person's history. Even the Yale Food Addiction Scale can be read as a description of someone reacting to their history of intermittent undereating, let alone strict dieting.[3] Ground zero for compulsive eating, these cofactors have not been accounted for in the food addiction research. Without teasing these factors apart, is it an error to arrive at the conclusion that everyone who claims they are a "food addict" actually is? Is it possible that a hyperresponse to food observed in the neuroimaging is simply the normal, healthy response if you are in a semistarved state—a condition to which career dieters can attest? This turbocharged reactivity to food can take place if you are, or have been, a highly restrained eater. Some people who vacillate between restrictive eating (dieting episodes) and periodic overeating—the classic stuff-starve pattern—show more physiological reactivity when exposed to food.

At the same time, megastudies demonstrate that many signs point toward stress relief and the reward system as what gives rise to food cravings, rather than the fact that you didn't have lunch. People who struggle to regulate their emotions are more prone to using hyperpalatable foods to soothe or distract themselves.

Needless to say, the food addiction research is in its infancy, and there are many unanswered questions. But the current research points to another solution that can decrease food obsession and eradicate compulsive overeating. Let go of dieting and start eating and living mindfully. By focusing on eating food that is not cracked out by the food industry to titillate your pleasure centers, you normalize your reward system response and reclaim the pleasure you can derive from natural foods (The Mindful Vegan Plate, page 116). Disentangle yourself from practices that distance you from living and eating with mindfulness: food and weight obsessions, tightly restricted eating, or a highly structured eating plan that disconnects you from your natural hunger and fullness signals. Support the shift with meditation, sleep, exercise, and connecting with friends. Now we're talking.[4]

Control vs. Acceptance Strategies for Treating Troubling Eating Behaviors

The dismal success record of standard behavioral programs—recall the weight-centric, behavioral approach we talked about in Big Diet—is largely because they don't adequately address *internal antecedent*. That means eating behaviors that arise in response to negative emotions that can generate food cravings. Here is where mindfulness, an acceptance-based strategy, has been more successful than control-based strategies. The mindfulness training implemented in the smoking-cessation program is an example of an acceptance-based strategy.

Control-Based Strategies—The Paradoxical Effect

Typical behavioral food and weight-management programs attempt to help you get a grip on your cravings and "addiction to food" with *control-based* strategies. Eat according to a strict plan. Remove unhealthy foods from your home and the office. Combat cravings by distracting yourself from them. Push away unpleasant thoughts and feelings that cause them. Shout those affirmations! This echoes the standard behavioral approach to quitting smoking in yesterday's lesson.

These methods have not been very successful, due to what is called the paradoxical effect.[5] Studies show that these thought-suppressive strategies *increase* the frequency, duration of, and preoccupation with the very thoughts and feelings they are trying to banish—right along with increasing the intensity of the distress they create. When the urge to eat a cookie arises and grabs your attention seemingly out of nowhere, trying to push away the thought that gave rise to the urge—or the thought about the cookie itself—is a difficult if not impossible task. It only leads you to grasp the thought in your mind all the more. When you finally can't take the tension anymore and cave, you are inclined to do so at an accelerated rate. In other words, you are more likely to plow through the entire stack of cookies, certain you're a sweets addict. Oh great.[6]

What if there is a way to interrupt the stress-reactivity-obsession process—so you can manage the stress reaction in a new and direct way?

Acceptance-Based Strategies

Unlike control-based strategies, *acceptance-based* strategies, rather than attempting to exert control over cravings and related feelings, approach them in a friendlier fashion through mindfulness. Mindfulness begins by increasing your awareness of your thoughts and feelings. Paradoxically, while accepting them as they are, you open up internal space around them to give you freedom of choice. This process relieves distress and increases tolerance of previously avoided or suppressed emotional experiences. Studies show that among people most challenged by cravings, the acceptance-based intervention is more effective in contending with cravings.[7]

Mindfulness Intervention

As an acceptance-based intervention, mindfulness interrupts the craving cascade in three ways: as your daily stress protection system, as your navigational tool for that moment between stress and emotional reactivity, and as agency for disarming cravings—should they already have grabbed your attention.

Daily mindfulness practice helps to keep you from building a towering wall of stress by helping you dissipate stress both during formal practice and through the course of the day. You start to see the entire stress train rolling down the tracks before it even pulls into the station of emotional reactivity.

With mindfulness, you become increasingly aware of your thought patterns. You recognize reactivity early on in your thoughts, feelings, and bodily sensations. If you don't know how you feel, it's that much harder to figure out how to deal skillfully with those feelings in a way that makes you more effective and leads to greater peace and personal happiness. Sometimes, we know exactly how we feel—frustrated by blocked goals, anxious about an impending challenge, or saddened by a loss. At other times, our feelings are a hopeless muddle, and we can only get so far as identifying how we feel as generally pleasant or unpleasant. Mindfulness strengthens your ability to discern more clearly how you are feeling in any situation. When it comes to changing from reactivity to response, awareness of the feelings that you are experiencing is crucial information. It helps you be more skillfully present, have more clarity about what to do next, and what, if anything, you should do about how you are feeling.[8] Mindfulness makes it possible to disengage from the obsessive thoughts that are craving's companions by interrupting the urge and reactivity autopilot.[9] This way you skillfully manage stress before it reaches the craving flash point.

Mindfulness also frees you from the angst of black-or-white thinking when it comes to favorite treats, as the process of bringing mindfulness to eating interrupts the emotional struggle associated with strong food desires. This frees you to eat moderate amounts of your favorites without triggering either guilt or binge-type episodes. Even if indulgence is already under way, with mindfulness you can reengage command at any time, interrupting the "abstinence violation effect" spiral.[10] Note I didn't say kick in the willpower. I said mindfulness.

We call ourselves food addicts and compulsive eaters, blind to the fact that continuing to see ourselves this way may well perpetuate the problem. If you've discovered, as did I, that this perspective isn't delivering, there is another way. Forming a healthy, happy relationship with food, eating, and your body isn't about never eating food for comfort, or banning your favorite desserts. It's about building a truly joyful eating and living experience that puts you back in command by giving you tools for connecting with natural hunger, navigating difficult emotions, and refurbishing reactivity. This delivers to you the keys to real freedom around food.

⚘ Mindful Moment: Wouldn't It Be Nice

"I am just not desiring the sweets like I used to. I think I'm losing my sweet tooth. Do you think it might be the meditation?"

During our first conversation a few weeks before, I had asked my client Carol, who was desperate to shed some excess weight and improve her health problems by eating a whole-foods plant-based diet, what she thought might be getting in the way of her success. Carol listed two things. First, she told me, "My moods dictate to me what I eat." And second, her overwhelming desire for sweets. Candy and cookies would call out to her just about every day, and she would be quick to reward the urge. I could hear the pain in her voice as she described the struggle to overcome the conflict between her healthy aspirations and her reality. Getting pulled into a craving cycle that is deeply entrenched is agonizing.

Within two weeks of starting mindfulness meditation practice, Carol told me that not only was the desire for sweets lessening, but there were fewer days when she even wanted them. Then, one day she grabbed a bag of her favorite candy at the market ("I deserve a little something!" was how she described her inner voice at these moments), and something different took place. When she got to her car and dove into the bag, she noticed that eating it simply didn't bring the rewards it used to. She had a few pieces, then stopped. Not because she was fighting the urge to indulge, but because the compulsion to eat the bag of candy had fizzled. Then, she surprised herself. She got out of her car and threw the rest of the bag of candy in the trash.

"Normally, I would finish the whole thing," she said. But this time, Carol was able to observe the desire for the candy as a thought. She even let go of the urge to "save it for later"—a big deal for someone who has a longtime aversion to "wasting" food.

Wouldn't it be nice if food just didn't do it for you anymore, in the way that it used to? With mindfulness practice, you get under the surface of these baffling behaviors that are making so much noise on the surface. Instead of trying to force something new, psychoanalyze why it is that you do certain things, or white-knuckle through what is troubling you, you discover how to work with disquieting states. With mindfulness, you find you can be present with tension, frustration, anger, fear, excitement, anxiety—anything that has agitated or unsettled you—so that these states can be dealt with directly or simply dissolve on their own. When we try to push these feelings away with thought, or avoid them with reactivity like cramming something in our mouth, we perpetuate their grip on our minds and hearts.

When I first began to have the kinds of experiences that Carol talked about, it surprised me. I didn't really believe that the pull of craving itself would be weakened in the way that it was. Instead of the usual hoping to win the war with an urge, I began to experience a feeling of emptiness surrounding what used to be a highly compelling behavior. This created a change. It began to happen just as Carol reported. An old food-related urge—the desire to make a batch of cookies and scarf down the dough—would arise. But instead of getting caught up in the fight, which was my usual next step on the cravings flow chart, something else would happen. At first, I'd go ahead and start the process as Carol had—the equivalent of buying the candy. But as I would begin, I would notice, just as she had, that something was missing. It was like an old boyfriend that you used to think you couldn't live without, but you now realize the thrill has gone.

From there, the process would be interrupted earlier on—before the virtual bag of candy was bought. Then, I'd notice the memory of the urge but realize how full of false promise it was—with a big load of pain on the back end. Ironically, we often deal with stress in a fashion that ultimately perpetuates it, seeking happiness in ways that simply lead to more misery. Lack of awareness and selective memory prevent us from being fully cognizant of the habits that are bringing us so much pain. The more we become aware of our own habits, the more easily we can detect which impulses cause misery and which don't. Once you really get that the hot embers grasped in your hand are what is giving you pain—and are furthermore practiced in the tools of release, as you learn with mindfulness practice—you can let go.[11]

This new view strengthened in direct proportion to being consistent with my meditation practice and how often through the day I mindfully connected with whatever was arising for me—whether mood, reactivity, or thoughts. This was a new way of being. I was becoming more aware of thoughts spinning and what bodily sensations were telling me about my state of mind and emotions. All without analysis so much as curious observation, kindness, and acknowledgment. Just as practiced on the meditation cushion.

During our initial conversation, Carol also uncovered the fact that she wanted, more than anything, a more positive relationship with food, eating, and her body. "If I could just keep a positive mind-set, as things come and go…" she would say. When we get right down to it, this is true for all of us. We want a better weight, a better body, a better…fill in the blank. Yet time and time again, I have found, as Carol experienced, that when we cultivate the positive inner relationship first, the ability to harmonize our actions with our aspirations becomes possible because we have navigated the part of the iceberg hidden beneath the surface.

We could keep whipping our dietary plan as in some Ben-Hurian horse race. We might win the race that way, but doubtfully the season. Even then we emerge with lash marks on our backs and blisters in our hearts and minds. The pain generated can be enough to drive us straight into the arms of our old pain reliever—food or some other distracting substance or activity—which provides instant relief simply because that is what we are used to. Followed by the misery of dashed hopes and self-recrimination, the pain can be excruciating, but at least we know how to deal with it. We're used to it.

I said to Carol on our first call: "Wouldn't it be nice if food just didn't do it for you anymore, in the way that it used to?" What if you could find a way that making the choices in alignment with your health goals and dietary ideal brought you more gladness than the previous injection of sweets? What if you became mindful enough of this process that you could see beyond the temporary tools you've been using—to something far more satisfying?

mindful movement

We walk our inner talk.

—JILL SATTERFIELD, integrative mind body counselor
and educator

Meditation Practice: *28 minutes*

DAY TWENTY-EIGHT, *Meditation on Breath and Bodily Sensations*

Physical therapy? Physical *is* therapy.

Physical activity itself can cultivate mindfulness and equanimity and dissolve stress. Today, you'll find out about another mindfulness meditation practice that isn't about sitting still, but rather about moving your body mindfully, shaking up your ideas about "anchor": walking meditation.

Movement and Mindfulness

Physical activity is the single biggest thing you can do to give muscle to the building blocks of the brain. Just like mindfulness meditation, exercise fosters neuroplasticity and neural connectivity, building a brain that can grow, change, and make sharper connections. As soon as you put the body in motion, biochemical events spring into action, stimulating the generation of new nerve cells that support many human functions, including learning and memory.[1] With both mindfulness and exercise contributing to the healthier, happier cause, what happens when we hitch them up together in more purposeful, concentrated fashion—in other words, with more mindful attention?

Movement-Based Embodied Contemplative Practices

All physical activity has some measure of mindfulness to it. You have to connect brain to body to climb the mountain, bike the trail, dance, or lap the pool. We know that one of the best ways to help children learn is to have them do physical activity while they are learning new mental skills—consider all the preschool songs accompanied by movement. This improves learning by better imprinting concepts in the brain. You have probably experienced yourself how activity makes your brain work better—the fastest way to shake brain fog is to put your body into motion.

In our overly cerebral lives, we have created a chasm between mind and body. In the West, we tend to see them as separate. This disconnect is reinforced by our culture, which gives lots of attention to what we do with our bodies and how to make them more fit on the one hand, and how to keep our brains healthy with various intellectual pursuits on the other. In contrast, Eastern medicine tends to see mind and body as integrated. Knowing how pivotal exercise is to better brain function, we can start to see how hardwired body and brain are.

The formal practice of mindfulness of bodily sensations opens our eyes to this intricate relationship of the mental and physical. Many exercise disciplines are specifically designed to enhance brain-body connectivity. There's a reason your mind feels so clear after yoga class. These are known as movement-based embodiment of contemplative practices. Tai chi and qigong are two of the best known. Feldenkrais, a movement-based learning method aimed at improving body-mind function, officially makes the list, too. These disciplines enhance well-being specifically because of the focused attention you give to movement of the body during practice. They ask you to be attentive and present, the heart of mindfulness. With seated mindfulness meditation practice, you anchor in the feeling of the breath, bodily sensations, and emotions, whereas with movement meditation your anchor is the feeling of the specific movements you practice during exercise. Dance, which requires cultivation of attention, physical sensation, and emotion regulation, and martial arts, with its emphasis on precision and attentive focus, beg to be included on the mind-body movement list. When you think about it, walking a tightrope, where one slip of attention to body placement can have disastrous results, qualifies, too. Perhaps the power that rock climbing has to pull one into mindful attention—bringing you right into the highly pleasurable mindful presence "zone"—is the real draw to the sport.

Mindful movement-based practices have resulted in measurable changes in physiological stress and improved attentional skills, cognitive function, physical well-being, and emotional states in healthy people. They have also proven to be effective for relieving symptoms of clinical conditions as diverse as cancer, Parkinson's disease, chronic pain, fibromyalgia, posttraumatic stress disorder, depression, and anxiety-related disorders.[2] For adults experiencing attention deficit hyperactivity disorder (ADHD) who find it impossible to sit still for traditional mindfulness practice, mindful movement practices can provide a good alternative.[3]

Walking Meditation

Thus far we've been doing formal mindfulness practice with anchor points of breath, bodily sensations, and emotions. There's another practice in the mindfulness meditation tradition that gets you off the cushion and into moving your body. It doesn't take any fancy equipment or skills. Just you, your legs, and your feet. And if you don't have those, you could accomplish the same thing with arms and hands.

Mindful walking is another way to bring more mindfulness of your body into your daily life. It strengthens your connection with all your body has to tell you, much of which we seem to be in the dark about.

Done in silence and usually at an ultraslow pace, perhaps the biggest benefit of mindful walking practice is that it helps bridge the gap between formal sitting and informal practice during the rest of your day.

Keeping the mind anchored and still while moving the body is not as easy as it sounds. As soon as you get your body moving, it seems your mind wants to start moving, too. After all, how often does it happen that when we walk, we are just walking? We're fussing over a project, planning the weekend, deciding what to make for dinner—even thinking about all the things we need to do once we've finished our walk. We usually walk with an agenda—whether that is to arrive at a location, get some exercise, or enjoy exploring nature or a new city. Usually, the ruminative mind comes along for the ride, too. With walking meditation, the difference is you bring your attention to the mechanics of walking and how it feels in your body while dropping other thoughts, just as the meditation on the breath is attentive to the feeling of the breath.

That's what makes mindful walking such a good training tool. It all starts with simply putting one foot in front of the other, with devoted attention to the sensations in your body as you do so. If reactions arise—wondering how this can possibly be of any benefit, impatience with moving so desperately slowly, the urge to hurry or get on with it—these give you the opportunity to work with reactivity. There's always a benefit.

You may not take to it right away, and it's not for everyone, so of course you can shelve the idea for now and try it at another point in time. But I found that my very resistance to walking meditation underscored its value. Once I got the idea and gave it a chance, I found I could bring more mindful focus to the rest of my day as well as to other physical activities, like brisk morning walks, bike riding, even scuba diving—enhancing the presence, enjoyment, and benefit of them all. And it can be a deeply delightful, in-the-flow-of-the-present-moment, mentally quieting experience on its own.

Walking Meditation Instructions

Find a place outdoors or indoors where you can walk ten or fifteen paces. This will be your walking meditation path. Implement the same steps as you do for sitting practice:

Position: Let your body be upright yet relaxed, your gaze slightly down and forward so that you are not in danger of veering into obstacles.

Anchor: Bring your awareness to the bottoms of your feet, and notice the feeling of your weight in your heels, toes, and balls of your feet. Even before you move one foot, you may notice your mind is off and running, chasing stories, toying with emotions. Gently shift your weight back and forth between your feet to help establish anchor.

Intention: Establish an amount of time for your practice. Just as in seated meditation, set the intention to notice each distraction with kindness, patience, and curiosity.

Remindfulness: Each time you become aware that the mind has wandered from simply paying attention to the sensations of walking, gently return your awareness to the feel of your body, on your feet, walking.

Now, take a step while keeping your attention as closely connected with the sensations of walking as best you can. Feel the lifting and placing of each foot, the extension of the leg, the shifting of your weight. Traditionally, walking meditation is very slow—it may appear to onlookers that you are in a zombielike trance. The point is if you move too quickly, it's easy to miss the nuances of the feel of walking, and your mind can easily loop into previous practices of going wherever it wills while you walk. Intentionally slowing things down is outside the norm, so it catches your attention. You can of course vary the speed or begin with a quicker pace before slowing it down. There are no rules except to find a pace with which you can be most mindful.

When you get to the end of your path, pause for a moment. Sense yourself standing. As you turn, feel the sensations associated with the shift of your weight, the turn of your body. Notice the impatience you may feel with walking so slowly! Observe the urge to do something else, anything else.

You will probably notice the dissonance of walking while actually going nowhere, as it is pretty much outside our usual experience. You can start with two minutes, or longer if you like. Walking meditation can also be implemented during your sitting practice time if you find yourself sleepy or restless, or the need to move is very strong, your mind distracted. It could be just what you need at those times.

☙ Mindful Moment: Spontaneous Mindful Awareness

As all your practices of mindfulness start to build upon each other, sometimes mindfulness will arise spontaneously, perhaps when you least expect it. Meditators describe this as being accompanied by feelings of delight, and a certain spaciousness characterized by ease, joy, and peacefulness in spite of what is going on around you. It's as if your mind is taking on a new skill without being prompted. In actuality, it is. These sensations and experiences of our own inner peacefulness are always with us. We've just gotten pretty adept at covering them up with our busy minds and fractioned lives. Learning how to return to them again and again is enough to change the entire quality of our lives.

DAY TWENTY-NINE

stress and anxiety

Not everything that is faced can be changed, but nothing can be changed until it is faced.

—JAMES BALDWIN

Meditation Practice: *29 minutes*

DAY TWENTY-NINE, *Meditation on Breath and Bodily Sensations*

Chronic stress makes us miserable. It locks our minds into a contracted state, sending us into endless rumination. It triggers a long list of difficult states, from a short temper to depression. Physically, it downregulates the immune system and negatively impacts our health.[1] In today's lesson we'll take a closer look at stress, expand the conversation to include her sister anxiety, and find out how mindfulness practice alters the profile of both.

Stress

Stress is the emotional and physiological tension that accompanies adverse circumstances, everything from traffic to a crash of your hard drive. Stress can have internal sources, too—our thoughts, negative interpretations of circumstances, catastrophizing, and other characteristics of the default mode network. It can seem as if we're focused on the negative, contributing to the stress load. We notice all the things that go wrong before we see what is going right. This negativity bias serves a purpose to keep us safe. We are hardwired to notice threats before the fun stuff. Knowing this helps, but it's not enough to solve a stress problem, whether acute or chronic. Mindfulness practice brings new discriminating skills. You learn to monitor your moment-by-moment experience so that you can step back from negative, distressing thoughts and feelings in order to view them as mental events rather than as unmediated reflections of reality.

Psoriasis Study

Among the first studies to test the effects of mindfulness on stress were conducted on patients with a stress-related condition—psoriasis. While stress is a well-known factor in the onset and severity of psoriasis flare-ups, few clinical trials for studying the effects of stress management on psoriasis had ever been done before these studies reported in medical journals in 1998.[2] In a pilot study, followed by a full clinical trial, psoriasis patients were divided into two groups. All the patients in the study were treated with the standard ultraviolet photo therapy. Those in the experiment group were also instructed to listen to a guided mindfulness meditation audio while undergoing treatment.

The results were profound. Patients who listened to the mindfulness recordings saw their psoriasis clear up significantly faster—almost twice as fast—than those in the group that did not listen to the recordings. Dramatic, considering that participants were only meditating between ten seconds and thirty minutes, three times a week, over the course of four months. And they weren't allowed to take the audios with them to supplement treatment with more meditation practice at home, either.

The results of these early studies led to the development of the now quite robust Mindfulness-Based Stress Reduction (MBSR) program developed at the University of Massachusetts by Jon Kabat-Zinn. Now in use at medical centers all over the world, this stress-reduction program is increasingly seen as a litmus test of how meditation can affect medical outcomes, including those related to stress and anxiety. MBSR directs participants to notice what is happening in their bodies and minds in the present moment, while either in seated meditation, engaging in a gentle movement-based practice, or lying down. In other words, just as you have been doing through the course of these thirty days.

Anxiety

Stress comes from life's pressures, as we are pushed by tasks, situations, even people (including ourselves), and undue strain is exerted on our minds and bodies. Adrenaline is released, and if it stays around too long or gets dumped into our systems too often, there's a physical and mental price to pay. Fallout can be increased blood pressure, insomnia, and other negative effects—one of which is anxiety. Anxiety is stress run amok.

Whatever the origins, anxiety is an emotion that none of us like. It is characterized by extreme discomfort and distress and can shift into feelings of sadness or depression. It steps up activity in the default mode network. Like being perpetually in a state of high alert, anxiety is about as far from being "at ease" as you can get. We all get anxious from time to time, and some of us have more anxious episodes than others. For some, anxiety is an almost constant companion, and profoundly disturbing. And we all wish we had less of it.

As with stress, understanding the crucial role anxiety has played in our evolutionary pathway gives us a little respect for it. It gives insights into how to navigate the challenges of anxiety so that it can do its job when appropriate and leave us alone the rest of the time. Our survival as humans has depended on our ability to be on high alert to the resources around us. Appraising everything from our social status to the changing weather and food availability meant a relatively constant state of the jitters. Step into your deep ancestral skin, and for a moment, think about how important being "tuned in" to your surroundings was for survival.

Whether it's acute or chronic, you can always find anxiety somewhere just below the surface, waiting to play its important role as your friend in the moment of need.

The results from the psoriasis study inspired more research to find out how mindfulness meditation—already long promoted as a way to reduce stress and anxiety—actually delivers when it comes to treating both. Soon another study was conducted on a group of highly stressed, anxiety-ridden employees at a high-tech corporation.[3] Subjects were randomized into two groups: one group completed the eight-week Mindfulness-Based Stress Reduction program, while the other group did not. Compared with the control condition, the mindfulness training changed brain function in specific ways over the course of the eight-week program. It produced more activity in the part of the brain associated with lower anxiety and more positive emotional states. Participants in the mindfulness training group also showed a measurable boost in immune function.

Mindfulness and the Stress-Anxiety Response

More than fifty studies now demonstrate that mindfulness-based programs reduce stress and anxiety. Several measurements, such as neurophysiological markers (heart rate, skin condition, fMRI imaging of amygdale activation) and the detection of hormone levels due to stress response, give us specific feedback. Self-report scales all point to positive results. In plain English, this means that cultivating greater attention, awareness, equanimity, and acceptance through meditation practice is associated with lower levels of psychological distress, including less stress, anxiety, depression, anger, and worry.[4]

Anxiety can be stirred up easily. A challenge to your ethics comes up in a conversation. An old struggle with food surfaces. Many, if not most, of our anxieties and fears come from rehearsing a possible future or rehashing the past. RAIN (page 134)—one of the cornerstone mechanisms of mindfulness—comes to the rescue again, bringing you into the present moment, quickly taking the edge off a high-anxiety situation. The moment you **recognize** anxiety is present (your body may tell you before anything else), **acknowledge** its presence. **Investigate** its presence in your body. What does it feel like in your chest, back, and shoulders? What is going on with your face? Can you feel the stress and anxiety in your emotional core, in your chest, stomach, and throat? Kindly and with compassion, navigate these physical reflections of an anxious state. **Nonidentification** allows you to step back from the anxiety, so you can see it as an emotional state that is arising and will in time pass away.

As your practice becomes more regular and you begin to gain insights into the changing nature of everything—including your thoughts, moods, and emotions—you can begin to see how to apply this same observation to the more difficult emotions of anxiety and stress.

Research is beginning to prove what mindfulness practitioners have known for centuries—that greater attention, awareness, acceptance, and compassion can facilitate more flexible, adaptive responses to stress. This in turn can help free us from stress-related misery and realize greater health and well-being. Research suggests that present-moment awareness of our thoughts, actions, and feelings during stressful events promotes our confidence to cope as well as act in accordance with our values—beneficial effects that extend into the next day. These results support the value of doing our best to maintain mindful attention during moments when we experience challenge and stress. Cutting-edge technologies, including brain imaging, are demonstrating the health benefits of mindfulness, an "inner technology" we all possess.[5]

While in the final edits of this book, I came across a new study that is a sign of just how interested medical science has become in the effects of mindfulness upon stress. In the clinical trial funded by the National Institutes of Health (NIH) aimed at measuring the ability of mindfulness to relieve stress, patients with anxiety disorders were studied. Significantly, blood-based markers of subjects' stress responses confirmed the stress reduction. Researchers discovered that patients who participated in a mindfulness meditation course had reduced stress hormone and inflammation following stressful situations. Those who didn't take the course had worsened responses. The control group that did not get the mindfulness training saw these blood-based markers rise.[6]

✿ Mindful Moment: Carolyn, Anxiety, and Mindful Eating

I have been a practitioner of meditation for several years. What draws me to meditation is the ability it gives me to control my anxiety. I have had anxiety since childhood and have used many methods to try and control it. Meditation affords me the ability to be centered, not only with the start of my day, but all day long. My morning practice is quite simple. I focus my attention to "just being there," focusing on my breathing. It is a time to rest my "monkey mind" and just be in the moment. My morning practice remains the center point of my day.

As a student of meditation, I am practicing being mindful of everything I do. I am mindful of how I treat others, how I work, and I am especially mindful of how I eat. I started with being mindful of my food preparation. This attention to my meals is what I call "mindful eating" [and] it is being in the present moment throughout the entire process. Even doing the dishes, I am being mindful of that process as well. For me, it has become a spiritual practice. It is a practice of eating "just enough" and enjoying each mouthful. I savor the flavors of the meal, much like people do when drinking wine. In our Western society, we are eating on the run—especially when we are stressed. It takes practice, but being mindful when eating can eliminate much of the "excess" we eat at meals. This approach toward eating has worked for me.

When I am "mindful" of eating, I enjoy the food better. I visualize and am thankful of how it was grown, and the workers who picked the food and prepared it for market. I am mindful and thankful for the ability to have fresh food sources, and I quietly meditate as I am preparing my meal. Before I found meditation, I just bought the food and prepared it without once being mindful of these other aspects of my meal.

In the past, I just ate the food without the ability to understand when I was full and when I was satisfied. In my younger years, I was a model and my thoughts about food were very unhealthy. I had a serious case of anorexia and bulimia. Having those conditions, and learning to develop a healthier attitude of eating, is really how I developed a mindful approach to food. My ability to foster a healthy attitude for my mind and my body really became the essence of my mindfulness meditation practice. It took work, but with practice and being in the present moment, I was able to change an unhealthy lifestyle. I have been on a plant-based diet for five years. With that said, not only have I been able to be an "ideal" weight, but I also have been successful in eliminating psoriasis, which has plagued me since childhood.

—CAROLYN LEPORE-DUKE, registered nurse,
health and wellness educator

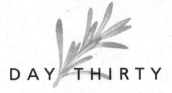

DAY THIRTY

a path with heart

*It is with our capacity of smiling, breathing, and being peace
that we can make peace.*

—Thich Nhat Hanh

 Meditation Practice: *30 minutes*

🔊 Day Thirty, *Mindfulness Meditation*

💡 "I'm really glad that you are writing a book on meditation," said Dr. Dean Ornish as we sat down in his offices near San Francisco to talk about *The Mindful Vegan.*[1] I had been eager to meet with Dr. Ornish, for of all the doctors who champion plant-based nutrition as important for better health, his approach is inclusive of meditation and mindfulness practices. In fact, as our conversation continued, it became clear that dealing with stress, increasing connectivity, and reversing our talent for disturbing our inner peace are the core around which all the other elements of the Ornish Lifestyle Medicine program revolve.

Your Innate Sense of Peace, Joy, and Well-Being

"We find that meditation is enormously helpful and powerful in a number of ways," Dr. Ornish continued. "Many people tend to overeat when they're stressed, as you know. A well-known food writer once told me that when she feels stressed or depressed, she eats a lot of fat because it coats her nerves, numbs the pain, or fills a void. Other things can fill that void, too—alcohol, drugs, working all the time, video games—there are lots of ways of dealing with stress, loneliness, isolation, and depression, which I think are the real epidemics in our culture. Meditation can help you deal with those stresses. The other nice thing about meditation is that you can see it not just as something you do for fifteen or twenty minutes by itself, but as an attitude that you bring throughout your whole day. You eat mindfully, for example—and then you get more pleasure with fewer calories. It is also really helpful in helping people create a sense of community where they can meditate and do these things together.

"It also helps you redefine where your sense of self comes from. I am glad to see that you are helping your readers understand that meditation doesn't *bring* them that sense of peace or well-being. It's not like valium in another form—it's already there within you. That's the whole point. We're born with ease and we get *dis*-ease, which disturbs that. When you meditate, your mind and body quiet down so that you experience more of your innate sense of peace, joy, and well-being. This idea is very different from what our culture teaches us—even the whole advertising industry—which is based on 'If only you had more whatever, just buy this thing and then you'll be happy, then you'll feel that sense of connection and community.' Once you set up that view of the world, no matter how it turns out, you're going to feel bad because until you get it you feel stressed. And we know that stress comes not just from what you do, but more importantly how you react to what you do."

Ultimately, it is far more effective to get to the underlying causes of the problems from which troubling behaviors arise than addressing the symptoms. We seek refuge from agitation, anxiety, and other unsettling states with a series of distractions. I shared my thoughts with Dr. Ornish.

"I agree," Dr. Ornish said. "You can tell people all you want that a plant-based diet is healthier for you, but if you don't deal with the underlying issues, the information about health alone is not usually sufficient to make lasting changes because these behaviors are very adaptive to dealing with the pain, alienation, and stress. If information were enough, nobody would smoke. The more you can address the underlying causes, the more powerful the healing can be."

Love Connection

A growing mountain of research underscores the compelling role that love, compassion, connection, and support—elements that vegan living, meditation practice, and mindfulness reinforce in our lives—play in our health, happiness, and longevity. They supersede and mushroom the benefits of healthy diet and exercise. People who feel isolated and depressed are three to ten times more likely to get sick and die prematurely from all causes than those who have a sense of love, connection, and loving relationships—including the one we have with ourselves—often independent of diet, exercise, cholesterol, genetics, and other standard risk factors.[2]

"Part of the advantage of a vegan diet is that it is another form of love," Dr. Ornish continued. "It's a love made manifest. Love yourself, love your family, love your community, love your planet. As we know, a plant-based diet is not only good for you, it's good for the planet. It frees up a lot of resources that can feed hungry people because it takes ten times more resources to eat a meat-based diet than to eat a plant-based diet, and more global warming is caused by livestock consumption than all forms of transportation combined. I've found that if these choices are meaningful, they are also much more sustainable. The nice thing about eating this way is not only is it the right thing to do for you, but also it helps a lot of other people. So often it's easy to feel overwhelmed by the crises. We think, 'What can I do as one person?' But when you realize that something as primal as what you eat every day can make such a meaningful difference, it imbues those choices with meaning."

A Quality of Attention

Our habit is to try to manage our experiences from a mental control tower, but through a filter of conditioning and reactivity. The stimulus-reaction cycle that we get caught in seriously binds our lives. Our freedom lies in responding, not reacting. This is a universal theme in terms of transformation. For each one of us, if we experience inner pain in any way, it is because there is some patterning that has locked in that we keep playing out over and over again, confining our sense of being.

Mindfulness invites us to take a different approach. It is about cultivating a quality of attention that you can bring to all of your life so that you can be mindful in the midst of your day, when a million things are demanding your attention. Through the mechanisms of mindfulness, you train yourself to notice the gap between the moments of an experience and your automatic reaction, awakening your capacity to open to a more skillful choice. This spells the fundamental difference between change from the outside in and change from the inside out. When we work from the perspective of the former, telling ourselves we shouldn't fly off the handle, white-knuckle through the urge to eat in reaction to stress, or squelch a desire to yell at the kids, it is like plucking the blossom off the plant. The blossom will just grow back unless we pull the plant out by its roots. Noting the gap between stimulus and response, you can unearth your inner wisdom and pull out the roots.

To realize a measure of healing for a situation, embrace and go through it wholeheartedly, with inquiry and desire for self-awareness. Otherwise, you surrender your ability—*response*-ability—to change things for the better. The result is dissipation of stress, reduced anxiety and other unsettled states, and increased emergence of your natural capacity for equanimity, calm, and happiness.

Mindful Moment: The Tuning Fork

Even in the midst of dismantling the British Empire's control over India, no matter how pressing the political situation, Gandhi would spend one day each week in silence. He believed this allowed him to quiet his mind and listen to the purest intentions of his heart, and act from the highest principles. If Gandhi—no doubt busier than most of us—can take a day, can we take a few minutes? Even ten minutes a day of mindfulness meditation, regularly practiced, can be of great benefit.

Looking back over these thirty days, what has been your experience? Reflect on any decreased stress, increased equanimity or balance, moments of peace or happiness, or glimpses into mindfulness as something that has improved your life experience in any way. Mindfulness practice is like a tuning fork, resonating our ethics with our work and our lives, freeing us from conditioned patterns by awakening a clearer mind—and a kinder heart.

day thirty-one and beyond

I T IS MY SINCERE WISH that you have found benefit in practicing mindfulness with me, and that your practice, and you, will flourish. There are many paths to awakening. Most of them, like mindfulness practice, include training your attention. If you find another way that works better for you, that helps you stay connected with your inner sense, I encourage you to grow that practice. Do those things that nourish you as a means of balancing and strengthening you. Spend time in nature. Move your body. Spend time moving your body in nature—a bona fide restorative.[1]

When you take care to do those things that cultivate balance and peace, you grow the resilience to allow yourself to respond authentically. Mindfulness is not merely about going somewhere and being peaceful, though it's wonderful when that happens. Each moment spent in mindfulness practice is important mental training that allows the emergence of your natural states of well-being. It teaches you how to live in each moment, with openness and less resistance, allowing your innate peace and happiness to shine. We can bring this awareness to any experience—whatever it may be. Even in the midst of difficulties, even in the midst of great joy, in the midst of anything—we can be fully present.

PART THREE

recipes

breakfast

dressing and sauces

salads and savory mains

sweet finishes

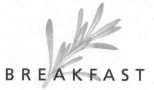

BREAKFAST

Mom's Baking Powder Biscuits with Almonds

8 TO 10 BISCUITS

This recipe is based on my mother's go-to for strawberry shortcake. These biscuits have since become a special breakfast favorite. I replaced some of the flour in the original recipe with almond meal, making it a little richer, cakier, and sweet. This recipe mixes up in two minutes and bakes in about ten. Can't find delicious any speedier than that. Thanks, Mom.

> *1½ cups whole-wheat pastry flour*
> *½ cup almond meal*
> *1 tablespoon baking powder*
> *½ teaspoon salt*
> *1 cup plant milk, soured (see note)*

1. Preheat oven to 450 degrees F.
2. Mix all dry ingredients together.
3. Add the soured milk, and mix until all ingredients moistened; avoid overstirring.
4. Drop by large spoonfuls onto a nonstick baking sheet.
5. Bake for 10 to 12 minutes, until lightly browned.

Note: *To sour milk, add 1 tablespoon cider vinegar to 1 cup plant milk in a glass, and let sit for 5 minutes.*

French Toast

3 SLICES

My search for a good vegan French toast took me through a series of unsatisfactory recipes that used mashed banana (too banana-y for me) or blended tofu (too heavy). Then one day I thought (divine inspiration?) to try tapioca flour in the mix. It added just the right crispness to the surface finish of each piece, and the garbanzo flour added more body to the batter as well as bumped up the bean protein. My husband, Greg, asks me to make this a lot.

> ½ cup plant milk (I usually use soy or almond milk)
> 1 tablespoon garbanzo flour
> 1 tablespoon tapioca flour
> ½ teaspoon maple or vanilla extract
> pinch salt
> 3 slices bread (I use a good grainy bread that I slice thickly, or
>   sprouted raisin bread)

1. Whisk or blend all ingredients except the bread in a flat container, making sure no dry lumps remain.
2. Heat a nonstick pan over medium heat.
3. Drop the bread one slice at a time into the liquid mixture. Turn to saturate both sides.
4. Place the pieces of soaked bread into the pan, and pour any remaining liquid over the top.
5. Heat each piece on one side for about 3 minutes, then turn to cook on the other side for another 2 to 3 minutes.
6. Serve with fruit, nut butter, maple syrup, or your favorite French toast toppings.

Sage Advice Double Mushroom Gravy

ABOUT 1½ CUPS

This is my new favorite version of my gravy go-to, recently updated to include a new find: powdered porcini mushrooms. I pack it with sliced mushrooms so it's nice and chunky—thus the "double" status. Your option, of course!

> *1 cup water*
> *1 tablespoon powdered vegetarian seasoning (see note)*
> *1 tablespoon tamari or soy sauce*
> *3 tablespoons garbanzo flour or rice flour (if you prefer a more*
> *   neutral taste), or a combination of the two*
> *½ teaspoon rubbed sage (more to taste)*
> *1 teaspoon porcini mushroom powder*
> *2 (4-ounce) cans sliced mushrooms, drained, or 2 cups fresh*
> *   mushrooms, sliced and steamed*

1. Place all ingredients except for the sliced mushrooms in a small-to medium-sized saucepan and whisk together. Bring to medium heat and cook, stirring constantly with a whisk, for about 3 minutes or longer, until the gravy thickens.
2. Add the mushrooms and stir to heat through. Serve over baked, mashed, or steamed potatoes; whole grains; steamed vegetables; or biscuits.

Note: In lieu of vegetarian seasoning, you could replace the 1 cup water with an equal amount of vegetable broth.

Lemon Cherry Salad Dressing

ABOUT ¼ CUP

With a pile of fragrant fresh lemons from my cousin's garden on the kitchen counter, I wanted to see if I could get a little creative and push beyond the squeeze of lemon juice on my midday salad. I had a jar of organic cherry fruit spread and decided to blend it together with freshly squeezed lemon juice using a mini milk frother, and it thickened into a tangy-sweet rosy whip. Tossed into my bowl of romaine, microgreens, garbanzo beans, and freshly chopped tomatoes, it was the perfect flavor addition, with just a little sweet to take the tart edge off the lemon.

On later occasions, wanting something a little more robust, I added a teaspoon of tahini and whipped that in, too. Perfect.

> 3 tablespoons fresh lemon juice
> 1½ tablespoons sugar-free cherry fruit spread
> 1 teaspoon tahini (optional)

1. Place all ingredients in a small jar or blender, and blend together.

Note: *This could be made with any fruit spread or jam, and with or without tahini, almond butter, or any other nut or seed butter of choice. If you like it sweeter, add a few drops of maple syrup or brown rice syrup.*

Turtle Beach Enchilada Sauce

ABOUT 3 CUPS

This sauce takes me back to the very first sea turtle project on which my husband, Greg, and I worked as volunteer field biologists in Mexico. We camped on the sand, patrolled the beaches to protect nesting turtles all night, and then collapsed on our sleeping bags at dawn. Needless to say, we were always enthused at mealtime to dig into the robust Mexican meals that were prepared for us. This is where I encountered the best enchilada sauce I've ever eaten. In my quest to find out the cook's secret, I peeked into the camp kitchen. Along with fresh tomatoes, some flour for thickening, and a wonderful bouquet of spices and seasonings, I noted three secret ingredients—chocolate, chipotle, and adobo. The flavor is complex, yet it's easy to make.

Here's my best attempt to replicate this sauce, going the easy route with canned tomato sauce. As a lazy cook, I take it one step further by letting my food processor do most of the work.

2 tablespoons garbanzo flour
1 tablespoon chili powder
2 teaspoons unsweetened cocoa
1 teaspoon chipotle powder (or more, if you like to turn up the heat)
1 teaspoon ground cumin
¼ teaspoon adobo powder, chili powder, or 1 tablespoon of the sauce
    from a can of adobo chilies
1 medium sweet onion, finely chopped
2 cloves fresh garlic, pressed, or 1 teaspoon garlic powder
1 cup vegetable broth
1 (15-ounce) can tomato sauce
salt to taste

1. Toss all ingredients into a food processor or a blender, and blend together.
2. Transfer to a medium saucepan and cook, stirring, over medium heat for a few minutes to thicken and blend flavors.

Note: *You can serve this anywhere you'd use enchilada sauce! With Easy Stack-and-Go One-Pan Enchiladas (page 259), as sauce on your rice and beans, or directly over a mountain of brown rice and red, black, or pinto beans on your plate. It also freezes well.*

SALADS AND SAVORY MAIN DISHES

Apple-Jicama Slaw

2 SERVINGS AS MAIN OR 4 TO 6 SERVINGS AS A SIDE DISH

Crispy, crunchy, and an absolute delight. Thanks to my sister Kristie for this recipe!

> *2 to 3 very crisp apples (same or different varieties)*
> *1 small jicama, about equal to the size of one of the apples*
> *2 to 3 small limes, zested and juiced*
> *2 tablespoons finely chopped fresh cilantro*
> *1 teaspoon agave or other plant sweetener*

1. Cut the cores out of the apples, but do not peel them.
2. Cut all of the thick skin off the jicama.
3. Julienne or matchstick cut the apples and jicama into a large bowl.
4. Add the zest and juice of the limes, then add cilantro.
5. Stir all the ingredients together. Add agave or other plant sweetener, and mix.
6. Taste and adjust by adding more sweetener, if desired.

Kitchari

4 SERVINGS

One thing I brought back from my trips to India is a love for Indian food. Kitchari is an easy-to-make beloved standard that brings all the best spices together in a fragrant bowl of comfort. If your spices are ground and not whole, that works well, too.

> 1 teaspoon whole black mustard seeds
> 1 teaspoon whole cumin seeds
> 1 teaspoon whole coriander seeds
> 1 teaspoon turmeric powder
> 1 cup mung dal
> ½ cup brown basmati or other brown rice (see note)
> 6 cups water
> 2 cloves garlic, minced
> 1-inch piece fresh ginger, grated
> 1 cinnamon stick
> 2 to 4 tablespoons fresh lemon juice
> ½ teaspoon salt

1. In a nonstick pot over medium heat, roast mustard seeds, cumin seeds, coriander seeds, and turmeric powder until the aromas start to mix and the seeds start to crackle and pop.
2. Add mung dal and brown basmati rice, and roast lightly with the spices.
3. Add water, garlic, ginger, and cinnamon stick. Bring to a boil, then cover and simmer for roughly 45 minutes, stirring occasionally, until dal and rice are cooked.
4. Before serving, add lemon juice and salt.
5. Serve in a bowl or plate over brown rice or other whole grain, with a few sprinkles of fresh chopped cilantro on top and lemon wedges on the side.

Note: *You can also replace the rice with another ½ cup dal if you prefer or plan to serve over rice.*

Easy Stack-and-Go One-Pan Enchiladas

2 TO 3 SERVINGS AS A GENEROUS ONE-DISH MEAL,
OR 4 SERVINGS WITH A SIDE SALAD

Desirous of a solid comfort meal but lacking the volition to spend lots of time in the kitchen, I pieced this dish together with simple ingredients that I usually have handy.

It's become a main-dish go-to. I've made this with my homemade Enchilada Sauce (page 255) as well as sauce I've bought off the shelf. It's very forgiving; you can throw anything that inspires you into the layers—olives, steamed vegetables, mashed sweet potatoes or yams, or stir-fried red peppers.

This quick-and-easy method of making enchiladas takes about five minutes to throw together, if you already have sauce prepared.

> 2½ to 3 cups *Turtle Beach Enchilada Sauce (page 255) or your favorite enchilada sauce, divided*
> 9 *corn or other grain tortillas, divided*
> 1½ cups (1 [15-ounce can]) *nonfat refried beans, or whole black or pinto beans, divided*
> 1 cup *cooked brown rice or cooked corn kernels (or both), divided*

1. Pour about ½ cup of the sauce into a large nonstick baking dish (I usually use my round, oven-friendly nonstick 14-inch Scan Pan).
2. Place three of the tortillas in a single layer on top of the sauce; overlapping edges is fine.
3. Spoon half of the beans in gobs over the tortillas.
4. Scatter half of the rice and/or corn over the top.
5. Pour another ½ cup or more of the sauce over everything.
6. Place another three tortillas over the sauce, varying placement so that it fills in some of the gaps from the first layer of tortillas.
7. Repeat steps 3, 4, and 5.
8. Cover with one more layer of tortillas.
9. Pour the rest of the sauce over the top.
10. Bake at 350 degrees F for about 30 to 40 minutes, until the sauce looks thick and glistening but not dry.

Note: *Serve as is or top with chopped tomato, cilantro, and a squeeze of lime to add brightness.*

Sweet and Sour Soy Curls

2 TO 3 SERVINGS

If you haven't yet had soy curls, here's a good excuse to try them. They are versatile, taking the flavor of whatever you mix them with, and have a pleasing texture.

1 medium onion, *chopped*
1 red bell pepper, *chopped*
1 green bell pepper, *chopped*
2 cups *sliced mushrooms*
1 cup *broccoli florets*
½ cup *vegetable broth, divided*

SWEET AND SOUR SAUCE

3 to 4 tablespoons *apple cider vinegar*
½ cup *pineapple juice (drained from can of pineapple chunks)*
1 tablespoon *tamari or coconut aminos*
1 tablespoon *organic ketchup*
1 tablespoon *organic unsulphured molasses*
1 teaspoon *fresh grated ginger*
¼ teaspoon *ginger powder*
¼ teaspoon *chili pepper flakes (optional)*
1 cup *vegetable broth*
1½ tablespoons *cornstarch*
half of an 8-ounce package *dried soy curls*
1 (20-ounce or smaller) can *unsweetened pineapple chunks, drained*
   (save liquid)

1. Stir-fry all the vegetables in the broth over medium heat, starting with a small amount of broth and adding more as needed. Cover and let these continue to cook over low heat while you prepare the sweet and sour sauce, checking and adding broth as needed to protect against sticking.

2. Combine the sauce ingredients and stir together until smooth. Then add the soy curls to the sauce to soak up the flavor—it will only take 2 to 3 minutes.

3. Add the sauce, along with the curls and the pineapple chunks, to the stir-fried vegetables. Raise heat to medium and cook, stirring, until the sauce thickens.

4. Serve over brown rice or other whole grain.

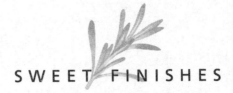

Chocolate Mousse

8 SERVINGS

I've come across several recipes for vegan chocolate mousse, but every one of them I've found too sweet or used large quantities of candy in the form of melted chocolate chips. Left to my own devices, I've come up with what I think you will agree is the perfect chocolate mousse.

> 8 dried dates
> 2 (12.3-ounce) packages of Mori-Nu Silken Firm Organic Tofu (see note)
> 3 teaspoons vanilla extract
> ½ cup cacao powder
> 2 tablespoons tapioca flour
> 1 tablespoon triple sec (optional)
> 1 tablespoon crème de cacao (optional)

1. Cover the dates with ½ cup of hot water and let sit for an hour or overnight.
2. Steam the tofu over boiling water (use a steam rack as you would for vegetables) for 10 minutes. Let cool.
3. Combine all ingredients in a food processor or blender and process until creamy.
4. Pour into individual dessert cups and chill for several hours before serving.

Note: *The secret to making desserts or cream sauces using tofu, I've discovered after much experimentation, is to cook the tofu first. This extracts any beany taste, and you'd never know that there is tofu in the recipe. I simply place blocks of tofu in a steam basket in a pan on the stove and steam them for about 10 minutes. This recipe also makes a fine chocolate mousse pie—just pour the mousse as prepared above into a prepared pie shell and chill.*

Vegan Cherry Garcia Ice Cream

2 GENEROUS SERVINGS

Who doesn't love chocolate and cherries in ice cream? This recipe is hard to mess up—it's always a crowd pleaser.

2 large very ripe frozen bananas (riper makes it sweeter!)
1 teaspoon maple or vanilla extract
¼ cup plant milk
1 cup frozen pitted dark sweet cherries
2 tablespoons vegan chocolate chips, divided

1. Slice the frozen bananas into ¼-inch chunks. If the bananas are ripe enough, they will be easy to slice and very sweet.
2. Drop the banana chunks into a food processor or high-speed blender. Add the vanilla and plant milk. Pulse until it starts to break down the banana chunks, then blend until smooth and creamy. If you need to add more plant milk, you can add 1 tablespoon at a time.
3. Drop the frozen cherries in and pulse only—you want to have big chunks of cherry in your final product. Simply mix as much as desired. If it gets too thick, you can always dribble in more of the milk.
4. Serve in bowls and sprinkle the chocolate chips on top.

Note: *As an alternative, you can add some of the chocolate chips after step 3 and pulse again before serving—they just tend to lose their chocolate flavor when frozen.*

Berry Good Ice Cream

2 TO 3 SERVINGS

My sister Pam whipped up this delightful creation, which delivers a wonderful creamy richness due to the avocado. Undetectable in the taste, it adds just the right amount of fluff and fats for a richer ice cream.

> 1 large frozen banana
> ¼ cup unsweetened vanilla nut milk, plus more as needed
> ½ to ¾ cup frozen strawberries (sliced) or raspberries
> 1 tablespoon chia seeds
> 1½ cups frozen blueberries
> ¼ avocado

1. Place all ingredients in a blender or food processor and blend together.

Note: *All the ice cream recipes can be placed in a container in the freezer for serving later. Depending on how long it is in the freezer, however, you may need to allow a few minutes of time at room temperature to make the ice cream scoopable.*

MANGO COCONUT ICE CREAM

1. Use two bananas instead of one, 2 cups of frozen mango in place of all berries, add ¼ cup of shredded coconut, and keep the chia and avocado the same.

resources

Now that you have in hand a dozen delicious recipes I've gleaned from my favorites to share with you, an important reminder:

🔊 *Audio Guide*

To support your practice, I have created an audio version of meditation practice to accompany each of the thirty days. Download free of charge at www.themindfulveganbook.com.

Navigate to Resources > The Mindful Vegan > Audio Guides. If asked, enter the password: freedom.

A few of these audio guides are available also for no charge on the Insight Timer app, available at insighttimer.com/. Navigate to Lani Muelrath and download selected audios for The Mindful Vegan Book Meditation Practice.

Forward, Together

I am interested in learning about your experiences with *The Mindful Vegan 30-Day Plan*. You are welcome to write to me at: lani@lanimuelrath .com.

For more information, speaking engagements, and mindfulness presentations for your group or event, please visit www.lanimuelrath.com and www.themindfulveganbook.com.

With love, deep appreciation, and hearty best wishes for your journey, *Lani Muelrath*

endnotes

introduction

1. Konstantin Batygin and Michael E. Brown, "Evidence for a Distant Giant Planet in the Solar System," *Astronomical Journal* 151, no. 2 (2016), http://iopscience.iop.org/article/10.3847/0004-6256/151/2/22.
2. Erika N. Carlson, "Overcoming the Barriers to Self-Knowledge: Mindfulness as a Path to Seeing Yourself as You Really Are," *Perspectives on Psychological Science* 8, no. 2 (2013): 173–186, http://pps.sagepub.com/content/8/2/173.full.pdf+html.
3. Ruth A. Baer, "Mindfulness Training as a Clinical Intervention: A Conceptual and Empirical Review," *Clinical Psychology: Science and Practice* 10, no. 2 (2003): 125–143, https://www.thehappinesstrap.com/upimages/Mindfulness_training_Baer_2003.pdf.
4. Margaret Cullen, "Mindfulness-Based Interventions: An Emerging Phenomenon," *Mindfulness* 2, no. 3 (2011): 186–193, http://www.margaretcullen.com/docs/MBI-An_Emerging_Phenomenon_Margaret_Cullen.pdf.

part one

1. Kieran C. Fox et al. "Is Meditation Associated with Altered Brain Structure? A Systematic Review and Meta-analysis of Morphometric Neuroimaging in Meditation Practitioners." *Neuroscience Biobehavioral Reviews* 43 (June 2014): 48–73, https://www.researchgate.net/profile/Kalina_Christoff/publication/261373893_Is_meditation_associated_with_altered_brain_structure_A_systematic_review_and_meta-analysis_of_morphometric_neuroimaging_in_meditation_practitioners/links/53e2625e0cf275a5fdd6efe3.pdf; Yi-Yuan Tang, Britta K. Hölzel, and Michael I. Posner, "The Neuroscience of Mindfulness Meditation," *Nature Reviews Neuroscience* 16, no. 4 (2015): 213-225, http://www.yi-yuan.net/Achievement/list_achievement.htm/pdf/pdf/2015/Tang_1426855548_1%20-final.pdf.
2. Catherine N. M. Ortner, Sachne J. Kilner, and Philip David Zelazo, "Mindfulness Meditation and Reduced Emotional Interference on a Cognitive Task," *Motivation*

and Emotion 31 (November 2007): 271–283, http://self-compassion.org/wp-content/uploads/publications/zelazo.pdf.

3. Daphne M. Davis and Jeffrey A. Hayes, "What Are the Benefits of Mindfulness? A Practice Review of Psychotherapy-Related Research," *Psychotherapy* 48, no. 2 (2011): 198, http://www.apa.org/pubs/journals/features/pst-48-2-198.pdf.

4. Britta K. Hölzel et al., "Stress Reduction Correlates with Structural Changes in the Amygdala," *Social Cognitive and Affective Neuroscience* 5, no. 1(2010): 11–17, doi:10.1093/scan/nsp034; Britta K. Hölzel et al., "Mindfulness Practice Leads to Increases in Regional Brain Gray Matter Density," *Psychiatry Research: Neuroimaging* 191, no. 1 (2011): 36-43, http://www.psyn-journal.com/article/S0925-4927(10)00288-X/fulltext; Sara W. Lazar et al., "Meditation Experience Is Associated with Increased Cortical Thickness," *Neuroreport* 16, no. 17 (2005): 1893–97, http://www.ncbi.nlm.nih.gov/pmc/articles/PMC1361002/; Antoine Lutz, John D. Dunne, and Richard J. Davidson, "Meditation and the Neuroscience of Consciousness: An Introduction," in *The Cambridge Handbook of Consciousness*, ed. Morris Moscovitch, Philip Zelazo, and Evan Thompson (Cambridge, England: Cambridge University Press), 497-549, http://www.psicoterapia-palermo.it/PDFS/Meditation%20and%20Neuroscience%20of%20Counsciuness.pdf.

5. Stefan G. Hofmann et al., "The Effect of Mindfulness-Based Therapy on Anxiety and Depression: A Meta-analytic Review," *Journal of Consulting and Clinical Psychology* 78, no. 2 (2010): 169–183, http://www.ncbi.nlm.nih.gov/pmc/articles/PMC2848393/; Abdollah Omidi et al., "Efficacy of Mindfulness-Based Stress Reduction on Mood States of Veterans with Post-Traumatic Stress Disorder," *Archives of Trauma Research* 1, no. 4 (2013): 151–154, http://www.ncbi.nlm.nih.gov/pmc/articles/PMC3876494/.

6. Marijke Hanstede, Yori Gidron, and Ivan Nyklícek, "The Effects of a Mindfulness Intervention on Obsessive-Compulsive Symptoms in a Non-clinical Student Population," *Journal of Nervous and Mental Disease* 196, no. 10 (2008): 776–9, http://www.ncbi.nlm.nih.gov/pubmed/18852623.

7. Elizabeth A. Hoge et al., "Randomized Controlled Trial of Mindfulness Meditation for Generalized Anxiety Disorder: Effects on Anxiety and Stress Reactivity," *Journal of Clinical Psychiatry* 74, no. 8 (2013): 786–92, doi:10.4088/JCP.12m08083; Michael D. Mrazek et al., "Mindfulness Training Improves Working Memory Capacity and GRE Performance while Reducing Mind Wandering," *Psychological Science* 24, no. 5 (2013): 776–78, http://www.ncbi.nlm.nih.gov/pubmed/23538911/; Michael D. Mrazek, Jonathan Smallwood, and Jonathan W. Schooler, "Mindfulness and Mind Wandering: Finding Convergence through Opposing Constructs," *Emotion* 12, no. 10 (2012): 442–48, http://www.ncbi.nlm.nih.gov/pubmed/22309719.

8. Viviana Capurso, Franco Fabbro, and Cristiano Crescentini, "Mindful Creativity: The Influence of Mindfulness Meditation on Creative Thinking," *Frontiers in Psychology* 4 (January 2013): 1020, http://www.ncbi.nlm.nih.gov/pmc/articles/PMC3887545/#B15; Brian D. Ostafin and Kyle T. Kassman, "Stepping Out of History: Mindfulness Improves Insight Problem Solving," *Consciousness and Cognition* 21, no. 2 (2012): 1031–36, http://www.ncbi.nlm.nih.gov/pubmed/22483682; Jun Ren et al., "Meditation Promotes Insightful

Problem-Solving by Keeping People in a Mindful and Alert Conscious State," *Science China Life Sci*ence 54, no. 10 (2011), http://www.ncbi.nlm.nih.gov/pubmed/22038009.

9. Sarah Bowen et al., "Mindfulness-Based Relapse Prevention for Substance Use Disorders: A Pilot Efficacy Trial," *Substance Abuse* 30, no. 4 (2009): 295–305, https://www.ncbi.nlm.nih.gov/pmc/articles/PMC3280682/.

10. Richard J. Davidson et al., "Alterations in Brain and Immune Function Produced by Mindfulness Meditation," *Psychosomatic Medicine* 65, no. 4 (2003); 564–70, http://www.ncbi.nlm.nih.gov/pubmed/12883106.

11. Barbara L. Fredrickson et al., "Open Hearts Build Lives: Positive Emotions, Induced through Loving-Kindness Meditation, Build Consequential Personal Resources," *Journal of Personality and Social Psychology* 95, no. 5 (2008): 1045–62, http://www.ncbi.nlm.nih.gov/pmc/articles/PMC3156028/.

12. Fadel Zeidan et al., "Mindfulness Meditation Improves Cognition: Evidence of Brief Mental Training," *Consciousness and Cognition* 19, no. 2 (2010): 597–605, http://www.psych.uncc.edu/pagoolka/cc2010.pdf; Heleen A. Slagter et al., "Mental Training Affects Distribution of Limited Brain Resources," ed. Mick D. Rugg, *PLoS Biology* 5, no. 6 (2007): 138, http://www.ncbi.nlm.nih.gov/pmc/articles/PMC1865565/.

13. Jason C. Ong et al., "A Randomized Controlled Trial of Mindfulness Meditation for Chronic Insomnia," *Sleep* 37, no. 9 (2014): 1553–63, https://www.ncbi.nlm.nih.gov/pmc/articles/PMC4153063/; Fadel Zeidan et al., "Mindfulness Meditation-Related Pain Relief: Evidence for Unique Brain Mechanisms in the Regulation of Pain," *Neuroscience Letters* 520, no. 2 (2012): 165–73, doi:10.1016/j.neulet.2012.03.082.

14. Eddy Larouche, Carol Hudon, and Sonia Goulet, "Potential Benefits of Mindfulness Based Interventions in Mild Cognitive Impairment and Alzheimer's Disease: An Interdisciplinary Perspective," *Behavioral Brain Research*, May 2014, https://www.academia.edu/27685650/Potential_benefits_of_mindfulness-based_interventions_in_mild_cognitive_impairment_and_Alzheimers_disease_an_interdisciplinary_perspective; Rebecca E. Wells et al., "Meditation for Adults with Mild Cognitive Impairment: A Pilot Randomized Trial," *Journal of the American Geriatrics Society* 61, no. 4 (2013): 642–45, https://www.ncbi.nlm.nih.gov/pmc/articles/PMC3666869/.

15. Diana Winston and Susan Smalley, *Fully Present: The Science, Art, and Practice of Mindfulness* (Philadelphia: Da Capo Lifelong Books, 2010).

16. Eileen Luders et al., "Enhanced Brain Connectivity in Long-term Meditation Practitioners," *NeuroImage* 57, no. 4 (2011): 1308–16, http://www.ncbi.nlm.nih.gov/pubmed/21664467; Heleen A. Slagter, Richard J. Davidson, and Antoine Lutz, "Mental Training as a Tool in the Neuroscientific Study of Brain and Cognitive Plasticity," *Frontiers in Human Neuroscience* 5, no. 17 (2011), http://www.ncbi.nlm.nih.gov/pubmed/21347275/.

17. Jean L. Kristellar, "Mindfulness, Wisdom and Eating: Applying a Multi-Domain Model of Meditation Effects," *Journal of Constructivism in the Human Science* 8, no. 2 (2003): 107–18, http://www.metanexus.org/archive/conference2004/pdf/kristeller.pdf.

18. Paul Grossman et al., "Mindfulness-Based Stress Reduction and Health Benefits. A Meta-analysis," *Journal of Psychosomatic Research* 57, no. 1 (2004): 35–43, http://www.ncbi.nlm.nih.gov/pubmed/15256293.

19. Evelien van de Veer, Erica van Herpen, and Hans C. M. van Trijp, "Body and Mind: Mindfulness Helps Consumers to Compensate for Prior Food Intake by Enhancing the Responsiveness to Physiological Cues," *Journal of Consumer Research* 42, no. 5 (2016), http://jcr.oxfordjournals.org/content/early/2015/11/17/jcr.ucv058.

20. Marcello Spinella, Sara Martino, and Christine Ferri, "Mindfulness and Addictive Behaviors," *Journal of Behavioral Health* 2, no. 1 (2013): 1–7.

21. Jennifer Daubenmier, et al. "Mindfulness Intervention for Stress Eating to Reduce Cortisol and Abdominal Fat among Overweight and Obese Women: An Exploratory Randomized Controlled Study," *Journal of Obesity* (June 2011).

22. Jean L. Kristeller and C. Brendan Hallett, "An Exploratory Study of a Meditation-Based Intervention for Binge Eating Disorder," *Journal of Health Psychology* 4, no. 3 (1999): 357–63, http://www.ncbi.nlm.nih.gov/pubmed/22021603.

23. Gillian A. O'Reilly et al., "Mindfulness-Based Interventions for Obesity-Related Eating Behaviors: A Literature Review," *Obesity Reviews: An Official Journal of the International Association for the Study of Obesity* 15, no. 6 (2014): 453–61, http://www.ncbi.nlm.nih.gov/pmc/articles/PMC4046117/#R31.

24. Jean Kristeller, Ruth Q. Wolever, and Virgil Sheets, "Mindfulness-Based Eating Awareness Training (MB-EAT) for Binge Eating: A Randomized Clinical Trial," *Mindfulness* 5, no. 3 (2014): 282–97, http://www.indstate.edu/cas/sites/arts.indstate.edu/files/Psychology/Kristeller_Wolever_Sheets_BED_In_Mindfulness_2013.pdf.

25. J Dalen et al., "Pilot Study: Mindful Eating and Living (MEAL): Weight, Eating Behavior, and Psychological Outcomes Associated with a Mindfulness-Based Intervention for People with Obesity," *Complementary Therapies in Medicine* 18, no. 6 (2010): 260–264, http://www.ncbi.nlm.nih.gov/pubmed/21130363/.

26. Scott R. Bishop et al., "Mindfulness: A Proposed Operational Definition," *Clinical Psychology: Science and Practice* 11, no. 3 (2004): 230–41, http://www.jimhopper.com/pdf/bishop2004.pdf.

27. Bishop, "Mindfulness," 230–41.

28. Ruth A. Baer, ed., *Mindfulness-Based Treatment Approaches, Second Edition: Clinician's Guide to Evidence Base and Applications (Practical Resources for the Mental Health Professional)*, 2nd ed. (Burlington, MA: Academic Press, 2014).

29. J. Mark G. Williams, "Mindfulness, Depression and Modes of Mind," *Cognitive Therapy and Research* 32, no. 6 (2008): 721–33, http://www.oxfordmindfulness.org/dev/uploads/Williams-2008-Modes-of-Mind.pdf.

30. Ellen J. Langer, "Matters of Mind: Mindfulness/Mindlessness in Perspective," *Consciousness and Cognition* 1, no. 3 (1992): 289–305, http://www.sciencedirect.com/science/article/pii/105381009290066J.

presence of mind

1. Jon Kabat-Zinn, *Coming to Our Senses: Healing Ourselves and the World Through Mindfulness* (New York: Hyperion, 2005), 108.

day three

1. Jon Kabat-Zinn, *Mindfulness for Beginners: Reclaiming the Present Moment—and Your Life,* Har/Com edition (Louisville, CO: Sounds True, 2012).

day four

1. Personal correspondence with the author, September 11, 2016.

day five

1. Felicity Callard et al., "The Era of the Wandering Mind? Twenty-First Century Research on Self-Generated Mental Activity," *Frontiers in Psychology* 4 (December 2013), http://journal.frontiersin.org/article/10.3389/fpsyg.2013.00891/full#B45.
2. Matt A. Killingsworth and Daniel T. Gilbert, "A Wandering Mind Is an Unhappy Mind," *Science* 330 (November 2010): 932, http://www.danielgilbert.com/KILLINGSWORTH%20&%20GILBERT%20(2010).pdf.
3. Q Li et al., "Abnormal Function of the Posterior Cingulate Cortex in Heroin Addicted Users during Resting-State and Drug-Cue Stimulation Task," *Chinese Medical Journal* 126, no. 4 (2013): 734–9, http://www.ncbi.nlm.nih.gov/pubmed/23422198.
4. Judson A. Brewer et al., "Meditation Experience Is Associated with Differences in Default Mode Network Activity and Connectivity," *Proceedings of the National Academy of Sciences of the United States of America* 108, no. 50 (2011): 20254–59, http://www.ncbi.nlm.nih.gov/pmc/articles/PMC3250176/.

day six

1. Judson A. Brewer, Kathleen A. Garrison, Susan Whitfield-Gabrieli, "What about the 'Self' Is Processed in the Posterior Cingulate Cortex?" *Frontiers in Human Neuroscience* 7 (October 2013), http://www.ncbi.nlm.nih.gov/pmc/articles/PMC3788347/.
2. Malia F. Mason et al., "Wandering Minds: The Default Network and Stimulus-Independent Thought," *Science* 315, no. 393 (2007): 393–95, http://media.rickhanson.net/home/files/papers/WanderingMinds.pdf; Brewer et al., "Differences in Default Mode Network Activity and Connectivity," 20254–59.
3. Judson A. Brewer and Kathleen A. Garrison, "The Posterior Cingulate Cortex as a Plausible Mechanistic Target of Meditation: Findings from Neuroimaging," *Annals of the New York Academy of Sciences* 1307 (January 2014): 19–27, https://www.ncbi.nlm.nih.gov/pubmed/24033438.
4. Kirk Warren Brown and Richard M. Ryan, "The Benefits of Being Present: Mindfulness and Its Role in Psychological Well-Being," *Journal of Personality and Social Psychology* 84, no. 4 (2003): 822–48, http://selfdeterminationtheory.org/SDT/documents/2003_BrownRyan.pdf.
5. "Meditation and Neuroplasticity, Five Key Articles," Meditation Research Psychological Science of Meditation, March 2014, http://meditation-research.org.uk/2014/03/.

6. Eleanor A. Maguire et al., "Navigation-Related Structural Change in the Hippocampi of Taxi Drivers," *Proceedings of the National Academy of Sciences of the United States of America* 97, no. 8 (2000): 4398–4403, http://www.ncbi.nlm.nih. gov/pmc/articles/PMC18253/.
7. Slagter, Davidson, and Lutz, "Mental Training as a Tool," 17.
8. Lazar et al., "Increased Cortical Thickness," 1893–97.
9. Brewer et al., "Differences in Default Mode Network Activity and Connectivity," 20254–59.

day seven

1. Yi-Yuan Tang and Michael I. Posner, "Special Issue on Mindfulness Neuroscience," *Social Cognitive and Affective Neuroscience* 8, no.1 (2013), http://scan. oxfordjournals.org/content/8/1/1.full; Sarah N. Garfinkel et al., "Knowing Your Own Heart: Distinguishing Interoceptive Accuracy from Interoceptive Awareness," *Biological Psychology* 104 (January 2015): 65–74, http://dx.doi.org/10.1016/j. biopsycho.2014.11.004; Catherine E. Kerr et al., "Mindfulness Starts with the Body: Somatosensory Attention and Top-Down Modulation of Cortical Alpha Rhythms in Mindfulness Meditation," *Frontiers in Human Neuroscience* 7, no. 12 (2013), https://www.ncbi.nlm.nih.gov/pmc/articles/PMC3570934/.
2. Candace B. Pert et al., "Neuropeptides and Their Receptors: A Psychosomatic Network," *Journal of Immunology* 135, no. 2 (1985), 820s–26s, http://candacepert. com/wp-content/uploads/2014/05/Psychosomatic-network-peptides-receptors-Pert-JI85-Pert-820-6.pdf; "Where Do You Store Your Emotions?" PhD, http:// candacepert.com/where-do-you-store-your-emotions/.

day twelve

1. "Binge eating disorder (BED) is marked by poor self-esteem, eating to handle emotional distress, extreme dysregulation of interoceptive awareness, appetite, and satiety mechanisms, and over-reactivity to food cues (Sobik et al. 2005) in amplified versions of more common patterns of mindless or imbalanced eating." Jean L. Kristeller and C. Brendan Hallett, "An Exploratory Study of a Meditation-Based Intervention for Binge Eating Disorder," *Journal of Health Psychology* 4, no. 3 (1999): 357–63, http://www.ncbi.nlm.nih.gov/pubmed/22021603.
2. P. K. Keel and T. F. Heatherton, "Weight Suppression Predicts Maintenance and Onset of Bulimic Syndromes at 10-Year Follow-Up," *Journal of Abnormal Psychology* 119, no. 2 (2010): 268–75, http://www.ncbi.nlm.nih.gov/ pubmed/20455599.
3. Heather M. Niemeier, "An Acceptance-Based Behavioral Intervention for Weight Loss: A Pilot Study," *Behavior Therapy* 43, no. 2 (2012): 427–35, http://www.ncbi. nlm.nih.gov/pmc/articles/PMC3535069/.
4. Michael G. Perri and Joyce A. Corsica, "Improving the Maintenance of Weight Lost in Behavioral Treatment of Obesity," in *Handbook of Obesity Treatment*, ed. Thomas A. Wadden and Albert J. Stunkard (New York: Guilford Press, 2002).

5. Heather M. Niemeier et al., "Internal Disinhibition Predicts Weight Regain following Weight Loss and Weight Loss Maintenance," *Obesity* 15, no. 10 (2007): 2485–94, http://www.ncbi.nlm.nih.gov/pubmed/17925475.

6. Ibid.; Meghan L. Butryn, J. G. Thomas, and Michael R. Lowe, "Reductions in Internal Disinhibition during Weight Loss Predict Better Weight Loss Maintenance," *Obesity* 17, no. 5 (2009):1101–03, http://www.ncbi.nlm.nih.gov/pubmed/19180064.

7. Tracy Tylka, et al., "The Weight-Inclusive versus Weight-Normative Approach to Health: Evaluating the Evidence for Prioritizing Well-Being over Weight Loss," *Journal of Obesity*, 2014, http://www.ncbi.nlm.nih.gov/pmc/articles/PMC4132299/.

8. E. Stice, "Risk and Maintenance Factors for Eating Pathology: A Meta-analytic Review," *Psychological Bulletin* 128, no. 5 (2002): 825–48, http://www.ncbi.nlm.nih.gov/pubmed/12206196.

9. Sandra Aamodt, *Why Diets Make Us Fat* (New York: Current, 2016).

10. Jean L. Kristeller and C. Brendan Hallett, "An Exploratory Study of a Meditation-Based Intervention for Binge Eating Disorder," *Journal of Health Psychology* 4, no. 3 (1999): 357–63, http://www.ncbi.nlm.nih.gov/pubmed/22021603.

11. Kristeller, Wolever, and Sheets, "MB-EAT."

day thirteen

1. Brendan R. Ozawa-de Silva, et al., "Compassion and Ethics: Scientific and Practical Approaches to the Cultivation of Compassion as a Foundation for Ethical Subjectivity and Well-Being," *Journal of Healthcare, Sciences, and the Humanities* 2, no. 1 (2012), https://tibet.emory.edu/documents/Ozawa-deSilva-CompassionandEthics-FinalPrintVersion-JHSH2012.pdf.

2. Christopher Hyner, "A Leading Cause of Everything: One Industry That Is Destroying Our Planet and Our Ability to Thrive on It," *Stanford Environmental Law Journal*, October 25, 2015.

3. "Assessing the Environmental Impacts of Consumption and Production—Priority Products and Materials," United Nations Environment Programme Division of Technology, Industry, and Economics, June 2010, http://www.unep.org/resourcepanel/Portals/24102/PDFs/PriorityProductsAndMaterials_Report.pdf.

4. "USDA Climate Change Science Plan," USDA, 2010, http://www.usda.gov/oce/climate_change/science_plan2010/USDA_CCSPlan_120810.pdf.

5. For extensive research archives on plant-based nutrition and health at the Scientific Foundation of Ornish Lifestyle Medicine, see https://www.ornish.com/proven-program/the-research/.

6. Dean Ornish, "Mostly plants," *American Journal of Cardiology* 104, no. 7 (2009): 957–58.

7. Robert H. Eckel et al., "ACC/AHA Guideline on Lifestyle Management to Reduce Cardiovascular Risk," *Circulation,* 2013, http://circ.ahajournals.org/content/129/25_suppl_2/S76.

8. Allison L. Crawford and Karen E. Aspry, "Teaching Doctors-in-Training about Nutrition: Where Are We Going in 2016?" *Rhode Island Medical Journal* 99, no. 3 (2016): 23–25, http://www.ncbi.nlm.nih.gov/pubmed/26929967.

9. Personal correspondence with the author, November 3, 2016.

day fifteen

1. Richard Chambers, Eleonora Gullone, and Nicholas B. Allen, "Mindful Emotion Regulation: An Integrative Review," *Clinical Psychology Review* 29, no. 6 (2009): 560–72, http://www.verksampsykologi.com/wp-content/uploads/2013/11/Mindful-emotion-regulation-An-integrative-review.pdf.
2. Norman A. S. Farb et al., "Minding One's Emotions: Mindfulness Training Alters the Neural Expression of Sadness," *Emotion* 10, no. 1 (2010): 25–33, http://mindfulnessmalta.com/user_files/2/neural-expression-of-sadness.pdf.
3. Chambers, Gullone, and Allen, "Mindful Emotion Regulation," 560–72.
4. Norman A. S. Farb, Adam K. Anderson, and Zindel V. Segal, "The Mindful Brain and Emotion Regulation in Mood Disorders," *Canadian Journal of Psychiatry Revue Canadienne De Psychiatrie* 57, no. 2 (2010): 70–77, http://www.ncbi.nlm.nih.gov/pmc/articles/PMC3303604/.

day sixteen

1. Shauna Shapiro et al, "Mechanisms of Mindfulness," *Journal Clinical Psychology* 62, no. 3 (2005): 373–386, doi:10.1002/jclp.20237.
2. "A Neurosurgeon Reflects on the Awe and Mystery of the Brain," *NPR Fresh Air*, October 7, 2016, http://www.npr.org/2016/10/07/496948795/a-neurosurgeon-reflects-on-the-awe-and-mystery-of-the-brain.

day seventeen

1. Bonnie L. Beezhold, Carol S. Johnston, and Deanna R. Daigle, "Vegetarian Diets Are Associated with Healthy Mood States: A Cross-Sectional Study in Seventh Day Adventist Adults," *Nutrition Journal* 9, no. 26 (2010), doi:10.1186/1475-2891-9-26.
2. Ciara Rooney, Michelle C. McKinley, and Jayne V. Woodside, "The Potential Role of Fruit and Vegetables in Aspects of Psychological Well-Being: A Review of the Literature and Future Directions," *Proceedings of the Nutrition Society* 72, no. 4 (2013): 420–32, http://www.ncbi.nlm.nih.gov/pubmed/24020691.
3. Juila Boehm et al., "Association between Optimism and Serum Antioxidants in the Midlife in the United States Study," *Psychosomatic Medicine* 75, no. 1 (2013): 2–10, http://aging.wisc.edu/pdfs/3006.pdf.
4. Ulka Agarwal, "A Multicenter Randomized Controlled Trial of a Nutrition Intervention Program in a Multiethnic Adult Population in the Corporate Setting Reduces Depression and Anxiety and Improves Quality of Life: The GEICO Study," *American Journal of Health Promotion* 29, no. 4 (2015), http://www.ncbi.nlm.nih.gov/pubmed/24524383.
5. Seanna E. McMartin, Felice N. Jacka, and Ian Colman, "The Association between Fruit and Vegetable Consumption and Mental Health Disorders: Evidence from Five Waves of a National Survey of Canadians," *Preventative Medicine* 56, no. 3–4 (2013): 225–30, doi:10.1016/j.ypmed.2012.12.016.
6. Aline Richard et al., "Associations between Fruit and Vegetable Consumption and Psychological Distress: Results from a Population-Based Study," *BMC Psychiatry*

15, no. 213 (2015), http://bmcpsychiatry.biomedcentral.com/articles/10.1186/s12888-015-0597-4.

7. S. Mihrshahi, A. J. Dobson, and G. D. Mishra, "Fruit and Vegetable Consumption and Prevalence and Incidence of Depressive Symptoms in Mid-age Women: Results from the Australian Longitudinal Study on Women's Health," *European Journal of Clinical Nutrition* 69, no. 5 (2014): 585–91, http://www.ncbi.nlm.nih.gov/pubmed/25351653.

8. Tamlin S. Conner, et al., "On Carrots and Curiosity: Eating Fruit and Vegetables Is Associated with Greater Flourishing in Daily Life," *British Journal of Health Psychology* 20, no. 2 (2015): 413–27, http://www.ncbi.nlm.nih.gov/pubmed/25080035.

9. Bonnie L. Beezhold et al., "Vegans Report Less Stress and Anxiety Than Omnivores," *Nutritional Neuroscience* 18, no. 7 (2014), http://www.ncbi.nlm.nih.gov/pubmed/25415255; Bonnie L. Beezhold and Carol S. Johnston, "Restriction of Meat, Fish, and Poultry in Omnivores Improves Mood: A Pilot Randomized Controlled Trial," *Nutrition Journal* 11, no. 9 (2012), http://www.ncbi.nlm.nih.gov/pmc/articles/PMC3293760/.

10. Gary C. Smith et al., "Effect of Transport on Meat Quality and Animal Welfare of Cattle, Pigs, Sheep, Horses, Deer, and Poultry," Grandin.com, December 2004, http://www.grandin.com/behaviour/effect.of.transport.html.

11. Felice N. Jacka et al., "Western Diet Is Associated with a Smaller Hippocampus: A Longitudinal Investigation," *BMC Medicine* 13, no. 215 (2015), http://bmcmedicine.biomedcentral.com/articles/10.1186/s12916-015-0461-x.

12. Bonnie L. Beezhold and Carol S. Johnston, "Restriction of Meat, Fish, and Poultry in Omnivores Improves Mood: A Pilot Randomized Controlled Trial," *Nutrition Journal* 11, no. 9 (2012), http://www.ncbi.nlm.nih.gov/pubmed/22333737.

13. Michel Lucas et al., "Inflammatory Dietary Pattern and Risk of Depression among Women," *Brain, Behavior, and Immunity* 36 (February 2014): 46–53, http://www.ncbi.nlm.nih.gov/pubmed/24095894.

14. Beezhold, Johnston, and Daigle, "Vegetarian Diets."

15. Balenahalli N. Ramesh et al., "Neuronutrition and Alzheimer's Disease," *Journal of Alzheimer's Disease* 19, no. 4 (2010): 1123–39, http://www.ncbi.nlm.nih.gov/pmc/articles/PMC2931824/; Kanti Bhooshan Pandey and Syed Ibrahim Rizvi, "Plant Polyphenols as Dietary Antioxidants in Human Health and Disease," *Oxidative Medicine and Cellular Longevity* 2, no. 5 (2009): 270–78, http://www.ncbi.nlm.nih.gov/pmc/articles/PMC2835915/.

day eighteen

1. Richard Davidson et al., "Alterations in Brain and Immune Function Produced by Mindfulness Meditation," *Psychosomatic Medicine* 65, no. 4 (2003): 564–70, http://centerhealthyminds.org/assets/files-publications/DavidsonAlterationsPsychosomaticMedicine.pdf.

2. Wiveka Ramel et al., "The Effects of Mindfulness Meditation on Cognitive Processes and Affect in Patients with Past Depression," *Cognitive Therapy and Research* 28, no. 4 (2004): 433–55, http://www.thaicam.go.th/attachments/362_R2010062803.pdf.

3. Farb et al., "Minding One's Emotions," 25–33.
4. Nicole D. Ottenbreit and Keith S. Dobson, "Avoidance and Depression: The Construction of the Cognitive-Behavioral Avoidance Scale," *Behaviour Research and Therapy* 42, no. 3 (2004): 293–313, http://www.ncbi.nlm.nih.gov/pubmed/14975771.
5. Farb, Anderson, and Segal, "The Mindful Brain," 70–77.

day nineteen

1. Kathleen Ho, "Structural Violence as a Human Rights Violation," *Essex Human Rights Review* 4, no. (2007), http://projects.essex.ac.uk/ehrr/V4N2/ho.pdf.
2. Marta Zaraska, "Mind over Meat," *Scientific American Mind* 27 (2016), 50–53.
3. Ibid.; Hank Rothgerber, "Underlying Differences between Conscientious Omnivores and Vegetarians in the Evaluation of Meat and Animals," *Appetite* 87 (April 2015): 251–58, http://www.ncbi.nlm.nih.gov/pubmed/25529819.
4. David Gal and Derek D. Rucker, "When in Doubt, Shout! Paradoxical Influences of Doubt on Proselytizing," *Psychological Science* 21, no. 11 (2010): 1701–7. http://www.ncbi.nlm.nih.gov/pubmed/20943939?dopt=Abstract.
5. Steven Loughnan, Nick Haslam, and Brock Bastian, "The Role of Meat Consumption in the Denial of Moral Status and Mind to Meat Animals," *Appetite* 55, no. 1 (2010): 156–59, https://foodethics.univie.ac.at/fileadmin/user_upload/inst_ethik_wiss_dialog/Loughnan_2010_The_role_of_meat_consumption_.._denial_of_moral_status.pdf; Brock Bastian et al., "Don't Mind Meat? The Denial of Mind to Animals Used for Human Consumption," *Personality and Social Psychology Bulletin* 38, no. 2 (2012): 247–56, http://www.ncbi.nlm.nih.gov/pubmed/21980158.
6. Gina M. Almerico, "Food and Identity: Food Studies, Cultural, and Personal Identity," *Journal of International Business and Cultural Studies* 8 (June 2014), http://www.aabri.com/manuscripts/141797.pdf.
7. Hank Rothgerber, "Can You Have Your Meat and Eat It Too? Conscientious Omnivores, Vegetarians, and Adherence to Diet," *Appetite* 84 (January 2015): 196–203, http://www.ncbi.nlm.nih.gov/pubmed/25453590.
8. Jared Piazza et al., "Rationalizing Meat Consumption. The 4Ns," *Appetite* 91 (August 2015): 114–28, http://www.ncbi.nlm.nih.gov/pubmed/25865663.
9. Nick Cooney, *Change of Heart* (New York: Lantern Books, 2011).
10. Sharon Salzburg and Joseph Goldstein, *Insight Meditation: A Step-by-step Course on How to Meditate* (Louisville, CO: Sounds True, 2002).
11. Gaëlle Desbordes et al., "Moving beyond Mindfulness: Defining Equanimity as an Outcome Measure in Meditation and Contemplative Research," *Mindfulness* 6, no. 2 (2015): 356–72, http://www.ncbi.nlm.nih.gov/pmc/articles/PMC4350240/.
12. David K. Sherman and Geoffrey L. Cohen, "The Psychology of Self Defense: Self Affirmation Theory," *Advances in Experimental Social Psychology* 38, no. 6 (2006): 183–242, https://ed.stanford.edu/sites/default/files/self_defense.pdf.

day twenty

1. Barbara L. Fredrickson et al., "Open Hearts Build Lives: Positive Emotions, Induced through Loving-Kindness Meditation, Build Consequential Personal Resources," *Journal of Personality and Social Psychology,*" 95, no. 5 (2008): 1045–62, https://www.ncbi.nlm.nih.gov/pmc/articles/PMC3156028/; Kathleen A. Garrison et al., "BOLD Signal and Functional Connectivity Associated with Loving Kindness Meditation," *Brain and Behavior* 4, no. 3 (2014): 337–347, https://www.ncbi.nlm.nih.gov/pmc/articles/PMC4055184/.
2. Christiane Wolf and J. Greg Serpa, *A Clinician's Guide to Teaching Mindfulness: The Comprehensive Session-by-Session Program for Mental Health Professionals and Health Care Provders* (Oakland, CA: New Harbinger Publications, 2015).
3. Jack Kornfield, "Loving Kindness Meditation," https://jackkornfield.com/meditation-on-lovingkindness/.
4. Shambhala Mountain Center, "The Science and Practice of Compassion," YouTube video, 1:07:02, interview with Kelly McGonigal, posted by Shambhala Mountain Center, October 22, 2016, https://www.youtube.com/watch?v=6BN9tAVQfQg.
5. Personal correspondence with the author, October 12, 2016.

day twenty-one

1. Personal correspondence with the author, May 9, 2017.

day twenty-two

1. Antoine Lutz et al., "Attention Regulation and Monitoring In Meditation," *Trends in Cognitive Sciences* 12, no. 4 (2008): 163–69, https://www.ncbi.nlm.nih.gov/pubmed/18329323.
2. Dominique P. Lippelt, Bernhard Hommel, and Lorenza S. Colzato, "Focused Attention, Open Monitoring and Loving Kindness Meditation: Effects on Attention, Conflict Monitoring, and Creativity—A Review," *Frontiers in Psychology* 5, no. 1083 (2014), https://www.ncbi.nlm.nih.gov/pmc/articles/PMC4171985/.

day twenty-three

1. Katherine Albro Houpt, "Gastrointestinal Factors in Hunger and Satiety," *Neuroscience and Biobehavioral Reviews* 6, no. 2 (1982): 145–64, http://www.ncbi.nlm.nih.gov/pubmed/6285233.
2. Elizabeth A. Bell et al., "Energy Density of Foods Affects Energy Intake in Normal-Weight Women," *American Journal of Clinical Nutrition* 67, no. 3 (1998): 412–20, http://ajcn.nutrition.org/content/67/3/412.full.
3. Sara W. Lazar et al., "Increased Cortical Thickness," 1893–97.
4. Personal correspondence with the author, September 30, 2016.

day twenty-four

1. Brown and Ryan, "The Benefits of Being Present," 822–48.
2. Gillian A. O'Reilly et al., "Mindfulness-Based Interventions," 453–61.
3. Celia Framson et al., "Development and Validation of the Mindful Eating Questionnaire," *Journal of the American Dietetic Association* 109, no. 8 (2009): 1439–44, http://www.ncbi.nlm.nih.gov/pmc/articles/PMC2734460/.
4. Ingred Elizabeth Lofgren, "Mindful Eating: An Emerging Approach for Healthy Weight Management," *American Journal of Lifestyle Medicine* 9, no. 3 (2015), https://www.researchgate.net/publication/273349293_Mindful_Eating; Christian H. Jordan et al., "Mindful Eating: Trait and State Mindfulness Predict Healthier Eating Behavior," *Personality and Individual Differences* 68, no. 1 (2014): 107–11, http://cupola.gettysburg.edu/cgi/viewcontent.cgi?article=1044&context=psyfac.

day twenty-five

1. H. J. E. M. Alberts, R. Thewissen, and L. Raes, "Dealing with Problematic Eating Behaviour. The Effects of a Mindfulness-Based Intervention on Eating Behaviour, Food Cravings, Dichotomous Thinking and Body Image Concern," *Appetite* 58 (January 2012): 847–51, http://www.thealegeland.nl/images/appetide.pdf.
2. Andrew J. Hill, "The Psychology of Food Craving," *Proceedings of the Nutrition Society* 66, no. 2 (2007): 277–85, http://journals.cambridge.org/download.php?file=%2FPNS%2FPNS66_02%2FS0029665107005502a.pdf&code=7dee7523cce0e0d6215d621ee092fd38.
3. Nicholas P. Hays and Susan B. Roberts, "Aspects of Eating Behaviors 'Disinhibition' and 'Restraint' Are Related to Weight Gain and BMI in Women," *Obesity* 16, no. 1 (2008): 52–58.
4. Richard D. Mattes, "Physiological Responses to Sensory Stimulation by Food: Nutritional Implications," *Journal of the American Dietetic Association* 97, no. 4 (1997): 406–10, http://www.ncbi.nlm.nih.gov/pubmed/9120195.
5. C. Nederkoorn, F. T. Smulders, and A. Jansen, "Cephalic Phase Responses, Craving and Food Intake in Normal Subjects," *Appetite* 35, no. 1 (2000), http://eetonderzoek.nl/wp-content/uploads/2015/03/nederkoorn2000.pdf.
6. Andrew J. Hill, Claire F. L. Weaver, and John E. Blundell, "Food Craving, Dietary Restraint and Mood," *Appetite* 17, no. 3 (1991): 187–97, http://www.ncbi.nlm.nih.gov/pubmed/1799281.
7. Kelly D. Brownell and Mark S. Gold, eds., *Food and Addiction: A Comprehensive Handbook*, 1st ed. (New York: Oxford University Press, 2014).
8. Yvonne H. C. Yau and Marc N. Potenza, "Stress and Eating Behaviors," *Minerva Endocrinologica* 38, no. 3 (2013): 255–67, http://www.ncbi.nlm.nih.gov/pmc/articles/PMC4214609/.
9. Kelly A. Gendall, Peter R. Joyce, and Patrick F. Sullivan, "Impact of Definition on Prevalence of Food Cravings in Random Sample of Young Women," *Appetite* 28, no. 1 (1997): 63–72, http://www.ncbi.nlm.nih.gov/pubmed/9134095.
10. Nicole R. Giuliani and Elliot T. Berkman, "Craving Is an Affective State and Its Regulation Can Be Understood in Terms of the Extended Process Model of Emotion Regulation," *Psychological Inquiry: An International Journal for the*

Advancement of Psychological Theory 26, no. 1 (2015): 48–53, http://dx.doi.org/1
0.1080/1047840X.2015.955072; Robert C. Schlauch et al., "Affect and Craving:
Positive and Negative Affect Are Differentially Associated with Approach and
Avoidance Inclinations," *Addictive Behaviors* 23, no. 4 (2013): 1970–79.

11. H. J. E. M. Alberts et al., "Coping with Food Cravings. Investigating the Potential
of a Mindfulness-Based Intervention," *Appetite* 55, no. 1 (2010): 160–63;
Kristeller, Wolever, and Sheets, "MB-EAT."

12. Esther K. Papies et al., "The Benefits of Simply Observing: Mindful Attention
Modulates the Link between Motivation and Behavior," *Journal of Personality and
Social Psychology* 108, no. 1 (2015): 148–70, https://pdfs.semanticscholar.org/cb0
5/6a2dee5cae2cb72fbd06be6c85ba3aa110c1.pdf.

13. Personal correspondence with the author, January 20, 2017.

14. Esther K. Papies, Lawrence W. Barsalou, and Ruud Custers, "Mindful Attention
Prevents Mindless Impulses," *Social Psychological and Personality Science* 3, no. 3
(2012): 291–99, http://doi.org/10.1177/1948550611419031.

day twenty-six

1. Paul M. Johnson and Paul J. Kenny, "Addiction-Like Reward Dysfunction and
Compulsive Eating in Obese Rats: Role for Dopamine D2 Receptors," *Nature
Neuroscience* 13, no. 5 (2010): 635–41, https://www.ncbi.nlm.nih.gov/pmc/
articles/PMC2947358/.

2. Paul J. Kenny, "Is Obesity an Addiction?" *Scientific American,* September 1, 2013,
https://www.scientificamerican.com/article/is-obesity-an-addiction/.

3. Judson A. Brewer et al., "Mindfulness Training for Smoking Cessation: Results
from a Randomized Controlled Trial," *Drug and Alcohol Dependence* 119, no. 1–2
(2011): 72–80, https://www.ncbi.nlm.nih.gov/pubmed/21723049.

4. Judson A. Brewer, Hani M. Elwafi, and Jake H. Davis, "Craving to Quit:
Psychological Models and Neurobiological Mechanisms of Mindfulness Training
as Treatment for Addictions," *Psychology of Addictive Behaviors: Journal of the
Society of Psychologists in Addictive Behaviors* 27, no. 2 (2013): 366–79, https://
www.ncbi.nlm.nih.gov/pmc/articles/PMC3434285/.

5. Rita Z. Goldstein et al., "The Neurocircuitry of Impaired Insight in Drug
Addiction," *Trends in Cognitive Sciences* 13, no. 9 (2008): 372–80, http://www.
sciencedirect.com/science/article/pii/S1364661309001466.

6. Sarah Bowen et al., "Mindfulness-Based Relapse Prevention for Substance Use
Disorders: A Pilot Efficacy Trial," *Substance Abuse* 30, no. 4 (2009): 295–305,
https://www.ncbi.nlm.nih.gov/pmc/articles/PMC3280682/.

7. Amishi P. Jha, Jason Krompinger, and Michael J. Baime, "Mindfulness Training
Modifies Subsystems of Attention," *Cognitive, Affective, and Behavioral
Neuroscience* 7, no. 2 (2007): 109–19, http://www.amishi.com/lab/assets/pdf/2007_
JhaKrompingerBaime.pdf.

8. Judson A. Brewer et al., "Mindfulness-Based Treatments for Co-occurring
Depression and Substance Use Disorders: What Can We Learn from the
Brain?" *Addiction* 105, no. 10 (2010): 1698–1706, https://www.ncbi.nlm.nih.gov/
pmc/articles/PMC2905496/

day twenty-seven

1. Johannes Hebebrand et al., "'Eating Addiction', Rather Than 'Food Addiction', Better Captures Addictive-Like Eating Behavior," *Neuroscience and Biobehavioral Reviews* 47 (November 2014): 295–306, http://www.sciencedirect.com/science/article/pii/S0149763414002140.
2. Philip Werdell et al., "Physical Craving and Food Addiction: A Scientific Review Paper," The Food Addiction Institute, 2009, http://foodaddictioninstitute.org/FAI-DOCS/Physical-Craving-and-Food-Addiction.pdf.
3. Ashley N. Gearheardt et al., "Preliminary Validation of the Yale Food Addiction Scale for Children," *Eating Behaviors* 14, no. 4 (2013): 508–512.
4. Ashely N. Gearhardt et al., "The Neural Correlates of 'Food Addiction,'" *Archives of General Psychiatry* 68, no. 8 (2011): 808–16, https://www.ncbi.nlm.nih.gov/pmc/articles/PMC3980851/; N.D. Volkow et al., "Food and Drug Reward: Overlapping Circuits in Human Obesity and Addiction," *Current Topics in Behavior Neurosciences* 11 (Mar 2012): 1–24, https://www.bnl.gov/isd/documents/77781.pdf; Harvey P. Weingarten and Dawn Elston, "Food Cravings in a College Population," *Appetite* 17, no. 3 (1991): 167–75, http://www.ncbi.nlm.nih.gov/pubmed/1799279; Andrew J. Hill, "The psychology of food craving," *Proceedings of the Nutrition Society* 66, no. 2 (2007): 277–85, http://journals.cambridge.org/download.php?file=%2FPNS%2FPNS66_02%2FS0029665107005502a.pdf&code=7dee7523cce0e0d6215d621ee092fd38.
5. Eva Kemps and Marika Tiggemann, "A Cognitive Experimental Approach to Understanding and Reducing Food Cravings," *Current Directions in Psychological Science* 19, no. 2 (2010): 86–90, http://www.psychologicalscience.org/observer/images/psychology_of_food_cravings.pdf.
6. Evan Forman et al., "A Comparison of Acceptance- and Control-Based Strategies for Coping with Food Cravings: An Analog Study," *Behaviour Research and Therapy* 45, no. 10 (2007): 2372–86, http://www.ncbi.nlm.nih.gov/pubmed/17544361.
7. Jill T. Levitt et al., "The Effects of Acceptance versus Suppression of Emotion on Subjective and Psychophysiological Response to Carbon Dioxide Challenge in Patients with Panic Disorder," *Behavior Therapy* 35, no. 4 (2004): 747–66, https://contextualscience.org/system/files/Campbell-Sills.pdf.
8. Lisla Feldman Barrett et al., "Knowing What You're Feeling and Knowing What to Do about It: Mapping the Relation between Emotion Differentiation and Emotion Regulation," *Cognition and Emotion* 15, no. 6 (2001): 713–24, http://affective-science.org/pubs/2001/01MaprelationDiffReg.pdf.
9. H. J. E. M. Alberts, et al., "Coping with Food Cravings," 160–63.
10. Kristeller, Wolever, and Sheets, "MB-EAT."
11. Judson A. Brewer, Jake H. Davis, and Joseph Goldstein, "Why Is It So Hard to Pay Attention, or Is It? Mindfulness, the Factors of Awakening and Reward-Based Learning," *Mindfulness* 4, no. 1 (2013): 10.

day twenty-eight

1. J. A. Zoladz and A. Pilc, "The Effect of Physical Activity on the Brain Derived Neurotrophic Factor: From Animal to Human Studies," *Journal of Physiology and Pharmacology* 61, no. 5 (2010): 533–41, https://www.ncbi.nlm.nih.gov/pubmed/21081796.
2. Laura Schmalzl and Catherine E. Kerr, "Editorial: Neural Mechanisms Underlying Movement-Based Embodied Contemplative Practices," *Frontiers in Human Neuroscience* 10 (April 2016), http://journal.frontiersin.org/article/10.3389/fnhum.2016.00169/full.
3. Dav Clark, Frank Schumann, and Stewart H. Mostofsky, "Mindful Movement and Skilled Attention," *Frontiers in Human Neuroscience* 9 (June 2015), http://journal.frontiersin.org/article/10.3389/fnhum.2015.00297/full.

day twenty-nine

1. Ronald Glaser and Janice K. Kiecolt-Glaser, "Stress-Induced Immune Dysfunction: Implications for Health," *Nature Reviews Immunology* 5, no. 3 (2005): 243–51.
2. Jon Kabat-Zinn et al., "Influence of a Mindfulness Meditation-Based Stress Reduction Intervention on Rates of Skin Clearing in Patients with Moderate to Severe Psoriasis Undergoing Phototherapy (UVB) and Photochemotherapy (PUVA)," *Psychosomatic Medicine* 60, no. 5 (1998): 625–32, https://www.ncbi.nlm.nih.gov/pubmed/9773769.
3. Richard J. Davidson et al., "Alterations in Brain and Immune Function Produced by Mindfulness Meditation," *Psychosomatic Medicine* 65, no. 4 (2003): 564–70, http://centerhealthyminds.org/assets/files-publications/DavidsonAlterationsPsychosomaticMedicine.pdf.
4. Jeffrey M. Greeson, "Mindfulness Research Update: 2008," *Complementary Health Practice Review* 14, no. 1 (2009), http://mindfulutrecht.nl/wp-content/uploads/2013/12/Greeson-research-review.pdf; Alberto Chiesa and Alessandro Serretti, "Mindfulness-Based Stress Reduction for Stress Management in Healthy People: A Review and Meta-analysis," *The Journal of Alternative and Complementary Medicine* 15, no. 5 (2009): 593–600, https://www.radboudcentrumvoormindfulness.nl/media/Artikelen/ChiesaSerretti2009.pdf; Paul Grossman et al., "Mindfulness-Based Stress Reduction," 35–43.
5. James N. Donald et al., "Daily Stress and the Benefits of Mindfulness: Examining the Daily and Longitudinal Relations between Present-Moment Awareness and Stress Responses," *Journal of Research in Personality* 65 (December 2016): 30–37, http://www.sciencedirect.com/science/article/pii/S0092656616301118.
6. Elizabeth A. Hoge et al., "The Effect of Mindfulness Meditation Training on Biological Acute Stress Responses in Generalized Anxiety Disorder," *Psychiatry Research*, January 24, 2017, http://www.psy-journal.com/article/S0165-1781(16)30847-2/abstract.

day thirty

1. Personal interview with Dr. Dean Ornish, Sausalito, California, October 13, 2016.
2. Dean Ornish, *Love and Survival* (New York: Harper Collins, 1998).

day thirty-one and beyond

1. Valerie F. Gladwell et al., "The Great Outdoors: How a Green Exercise Environment Can Benefit All," *Extreme Physiology and Medicine* 2, no. 3 (2013), https://www.ncbi.nlm.nih.gov/pmc/articles/PMC3710158/.

index

acknowledgments

To the many who have contributed to this book through personal interview, I am grateful to each of you for opening your hearts, minds, and office doors to me. Dean Ornish, what a delightful surprise to find so much common ground—it's not just the food; it's the whole person—thank you for your hearty enthusiasm for *The Mindful Vegan*. Judson Brewer, neuroscientist extraordinaire, thank you for sharing your expertise at connecting the dots between neuroscience and the mindfulness experience—it's endlessly fascinating. Melanie Joy, your brilliance at connecting compassion with common sense is deeply appreciated, and I treasure our friendship and your contributions to this book. Brenda Davis, thank you for putting your five-star approval on the nutrition sections and your unbridled enthusiasm for the topic of this book. I consider myself deeply fortunate to have the support of such an enlightened dietitian. Special thanks to Patti Breitman, and Will Tuttle—advocates and activists leading the way.

To my mindfulness meditation teachers, each of you has tremendously impacted my personal practice, my work, and my life, notably S. N. Goenka, Diana Winston, Jack Kornfield, Jill Satterfield, Heather Sundberg, and many others who have provided instruction and insight along the way.

Neal Barnard, your zeal for and devotion to conscious eating continues to impress me and the world. You are a true leader for our times. Thank you for your friendship, encouragement, and kind, generous offer to contribute the brilliant foreword for *The Mindful Vegan*.

For your contributions and shining support, heartfelt thanks to Jean Antonello, Nick Cooney, Bethany Davis, Carolyn Lepore-Duke, Karenna Love, Sharon McRae, Ari Nessel, Nina Osberg, Marla Rose, Miyoko Schinner, Kathryn Stafford, and Wendy Werneth. Thank you to my parents, Dorothy and Chet Younghans. Mom, thank you for modeling the search for truth and for teaching me the value of quiet introspection.

To my recipe testers: Brandie Bloggins, Cheryl Duvall, Charlie Fields, Kristie Foss, Andrea Ivins, Sybil Janke, Kim Logan, Liz McCarthy, Lori Pratley, Catherine Rehm, Amy Shockley, Allie Shockley, Christine Vitale, and Pam Younghans. Thank you for sharing your creations and for diving into the recipes with curiosity and enthusiasm—and making them even better!

Deep appreciation and thanks to my darling husband, Greg, the love of my life, for your support through the ups, downs, demands, and various nuances of an author's life.

Thanks to my literary agent, Marilyn Allen, for your vision, passion for, and confidence in this project. To everyone at BenBella Books—Glenn Yeffeth, Heather Butterfield, Sarah Dombrowsky, Alicia Kania, Adrienne Lang, Lindsay Marshall, Monica Lowry, and Vy Tran, thank you for your expertise, excitement, and enthusiasm for *The Mindful Vegan*—Her time has come.

about the author

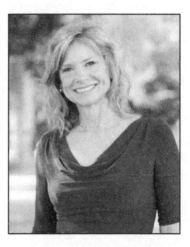

LANI MUELRATH, MA, is an award-winning health educator, best-selling author, inspirational speaker, and TV host widely sought for her expertise in plant-based, vegan, active, mindful living. Lani has been featured on CBS-TV, ABC-TV, *Prevention* magazine, *USA Today*, the *Saturday Evening Post*, and NSPR. She created and starred in her own CBS television show, *Lani's All-Heart Aerobics*, and has served as presenter and consultant for the Physician's Committee for Responsible Medicine, the Complete Health Improvement Project, and Plant Pure Nation.

Lani has been vegetarian/vegan for forty-five years and has been teaching in health and wellness for over four decades. She has practiced mindfulness meditation for over twenty-five years. Recognized as a thought leader and pioneer in the integration of vegan living, fitness, and mindfulness, Lani's approach blends plant-based nutrition with compassion, mind/body awareness, movement, and transformational techniques from mindfulness meditation practice.

Certified in Mindfulness Meditation Instruction, and in Plant-Based Nutrition from Cornell University, Lani is also an authorized Mind-body Specialist and Behavior Change Specialist. Her multiple teaching credentials include Yoga, Physical Education, and Advanced Fitness Nutrition. The recipient of the California Golden Apple Award for Excellence in Instruction, Lani has been guest lecturer at San Francisco State University and is associate faculty in Kinesiology at Butte College, where one of her books has been adopted as required text.

The Mindful Vegan is Lani's third book, following *The Plant-Based Journey: A Step-By-Step Guide for Transitioning to a Healthy Lifestyle and Achieving Your Ideal Weight*, awarded Top Media Pick by *VegNews* magazine, and *Fit Quickies: 5 Minute Targeted Body-Shaping Workouts*.

Lani lives in the Sierra/Cascade foothills in Northern California with her husband, Greg, with whom she travels the world on wildlife advocacy missions and scuba, hiking, and bicycling adventures.

Join Lani's community at LaniMuelrath.com and on social media:

Facebook: lanimuelrath

Instagram: lani.muelrath

Twitter: @lanimuelrath